What Paramedics Should Know

Copyright

What Paramedics Should Know

Steven M Morken

CONTENTS

This book wouldn't exist without the countless individuals who have shaped my journey as a paramedic and, by extension, this narrative. First and foremost, I owe a debt of gratitude to my colleagues – the unsung heroes who share the highs and lows of this demanding profession. Their stories, both spoken and unspoken, are woven into the fabric of these pages. I'm particularly grateful to Sarah Chen, whose unwavering support and insightful feedback were invaluable during the writing process. Her willingness to share her own experiences brought a crucial dimension of authenticity to the text. A special thanks also goes to the patients, families, and communities I've served throughout my career. Your resilience and strength have continually inspired me. Finally, to my family – your patience and understanding have been my unwavering anchor. This book is as much a testament to your sacrifices as it is to the experiences within.

The Siren's Call: Why We Chose This Life

The siren's song, for many, is a call to heroism, a potent blend of adrenaline and altruism. It whispers promises of making a difference, of being the one to arrive when seconds count, of saving lives in moments of extreme crisis. This idealism, vibrant and unwavering, is often the very force that drives aspiring paramedics through the grueling crucible of training. I remember it well, that initial fire, that fervent belief in my own potential to become a beacon of hope in the face of unimaginable suffering. My application, filled out with the nervous energy of a seasoned marathon runner just before the starting gun, spoke volumes of this untested conviction.

But the reality of paramedic training often shatters that pristine vision. The academy, a seemingly innocuous word, transforms into a battlefield of exhaustion, frustration, and self-doubt. The initial euphoria gives way to a relentless barrage of challenges, both physical and mental. The sheer volume of information to absorb—anatomy, physiology, pharmacology, countless emergency procedures—is overwhelming. The seemingly endless practical sessions, often conducted in simulated environments mirroring the chaos of real-world emergencies, become a grueling test of endurance. Imagine a relentless fire hose of knowledge directed at you, forcing you to retain every drop, to absorb and process it all before the next wave crashes down.

For example, the sheer physical toll of the training is something that many fail to anticipate. Hours spent practicing CPR, moving heavy patients on stretchers, and navigating obstacle courses designed to replicate the demanding physical labor of the job. My own body ached constantly; muscles I never knew existed screamed in protest. The sleep deprivation alone was enough to fray the nerves, let alone the accumulated mental strain. The pressure mounts with every failed practical assessment, every missed detail in an intricate scenario that could represent a life or death situation in the field. I remember one particular scenario where we were training on managing a multiple casualty incident and the sheer chaos of juggling simulated injuries across multiple victims pushed me to my absolute limit.

The mental fortitude required is perhaps even more demanding. The relentless pressure to perform flawlessly, the constant exposure to simulated trauma, and the unwavering expectation of proficiency leave many feeling emotionally drained and mentally exhausted. The emotional landscape of training is far from idyllic; the constant exposure to simulated death and suffering can take a heavy toll. We were tasked with managing simulated scenarios involving child trauma and responding to simulated calls of domestic violence and the emotional residue of these experiences is significant even in the artificial construct of training. The academy becomes a crucible, forging resilience in some but shattering the dreams of others. I watched friends, some initially equally enthusiastic, falter and withdraw, their idealism slowly eroded by the relentless demands.

Beyond the sheer volume of knowledge and skills to master, the pressure to perform is relentless. Each practical assessment, each written exam, is a high-stakes event, the pressure magnified by the knowledge that one slip-up could mean failure and the abandonment of a cherished dream. This isn't a mere academic exercise; it is the preparation for a career where mistakes can have devastating consequences. The consequences for failure extend beyond a simple failing grade; it is the potential to fail a patient and the immense weight of that possibility that drives the tension.

Furthermore, the intense competitive environment within the academy can add another layer of pressure. While collaboration and team-work are essential, there's an underlying sense of competition for limited spots in the field training program and ultimately, a limited number of paramedic positions. Every assessment becomes a race, where those who lack the resilience to overcome the intense pressure are weeded out. It's a system designed to select only the most resilient and capable candidates.

However, it's not solely a story of struggle. The challenges are not insurmountable; they are, in fact, integral to the process. The academy isn't merely designed to weed out the weak but rather to cultivate strength, resilience, and a deeper understanding of what it truly means to be a paramedic. The camaraderie forged amongst the trainees in the face of adversity, the unwavering support of instructors who have walked this difficult path, and the profound sense of shared purpose can create an unbreakable bond that will be invaluable throughout a paramedic's career.

The shared hardships create a unique bond between classmates. The exhaustion, the frustrations, the shared triumphs become stories that unite us and serve as a foundation for the professional relationships we form in the field. I still remember late-night study sessions fueled by lukewarm coffee and sheer determination, the quiet moments of mutual support when one of us felt overwhelmed, the celebration that followed a particularly challenging practical assessment. These relationships transcended the classroom. Many of these fellow students remain amongst my closest confidants, a reminder of the difficult path we've all shared.

The instructors, seasoned professionals who have witnessed the highs and lows of this profession, play a vital role. Their guidance, not only in technical skills but in emotional resilience, is invaluable. Their willingness to share not only the technicalities of the job but their own experiences, the difficult calls, and the emotional scars, is what separates truly excellent instructors from the rest. They served not just as teachers but as mentors, helping us to navigate the emotional roller coaster of training and preparing us for the profound emotional toll the job demands.

The process of overcoming these challenges shapes the paramedic. The resilience forged in the crucible of training isn't just about physical strength; it's about mental toughness, the ability to remain calm under pressure, the clarity to make critical decisions under immense stress. It's about the ability to compartmentalize the trauma, to process the emotional impact without succumbing to its weight. This isn't a skill taught in a textbook; it is a skill honed through experience, both simulated and real.

So, the initial idealism of the aspiring paramedic is not misplaced. It is, in fact, the essential fuel that propels them through the rigors of training. However, the training itself is a necessary process, one that strips away the naivete, replaces it with grit, and molds the idealistic novice into a resilient, resourceful, and compassionate professional. The transformation is profound, and it is a testament to the strength and dedication of those who persevere. The experience is not without its scars, emotional and physical, yet ultimately it forges a foundation of skill, resilience and empathy upon which a successful career can be built. The journey from idealistic student to seasoned paramedic is long and arduous but for those who persevere, the reward is a life dedicated to service, healing, and a profound understanding of human resilience in the face of suffering.

The siren's call, answered with such fervent idealism, leads us to a reality far more intricate than the initial romanticized vision. While the initial training focuses on the adrenaline-fueled drama, the true foundation of a paramedic's success lies in a deep and comprehensive understanding of the human body, its vulnerabilities, and its remarkable capacity for resilience. This understanding, meticulously built upon years of study and honed through countless hours of practice, forms the bedrock of our ability to assess, treat, and ultimately, save lives.

Anatomy, the very blueprint of the human form, is our first and most fundamental tool. It's not just rote memorization of bone names and muscle origins; it's about understanding the intricate interplay of systems, the cascading effects of injury, and the subtle signs that often betray the severity of a condition. Knowing the precise location of major blood vessels is crucial not only for effective intravenous access but also for anticipating the potential for life-threatening hemorrhage. Similarly, a thorough understanding of the respiratory system allows us to interpret subtle changes in breathing patterns, recognizing the signs of impending respiratory failure.

I remember one particularly harrowing call where an elderly woman was found unconscious in her home. My initial assessment revealed no obvious external injuries, but her shallow, irregular breathing hinted at a more serious underlying issue. A comprehensive understanding of the anatomy of the lungs, trachea, and surrounding structures allowed me to recognize the subtleties of her breathing pattern. It immediately raised suspicion of a pulmonary embolism, a life-threatening blood clot in the lungs, and the subsequent rapid assessment and interventions saved her life. The knowledge was not just a checklist; it was intuitive understanding guiding decision-making in the face of extreme pressure.

Beyond anatomy, physiology provides the dynamic context. It's understanding not just *what* is there, but *how* it works, how systems interact, and how they respond to injury or disease. This understanding is not just theoretical; it is the key to interpreting vital signs, understanding the body's compensatory mechanisms, and predicting the potential trajectory of a patient's condition. A simple tachycardia (rapid heart rate) can be a sign of many things; the underlying physiology guides us towards the correct diagnosis, whether it be hypovolemia (low blood volume), anxiety, or a cardiac event. Knowing *why* the body responds in certain ways is what allows us to anticipate complications and make informed clinical decisions.

Pharmacology, the study of drugs, is another critical pillar. It's more than just knowing the names of medications and their indications; it's about understanding their mechanisms of action, their potential side effects, and their interactions with other drugs. In the high-pressure environment of an emergency call, administering the wrong medication, or the wrong dose, can have disastrous consequences. I've seen firsthand the devastating impact of a simple medication error, and the memory serves as a constant reminder of the importance of precision and meticulous attention to detail. A thorough grasp of pharmacology doesn't just prevent mistakes; it enables us to tailor treatment to the specific needs of the patient, optimizing their chance of survival and recovery.

Beyond the core sciences, procedural skills are paramount. Intra-venous cannulation, an essential skill for administering medications and fluids, requires precision and a steady hand. It's not just about finding the vein; it's about assessing the patient's overall condition, choosing the appropriate site, and performing the procedure with minimal discomfort and risk of complications. Similarly, advanced airway management—intubation and other advanced airway techniques—demands both technical proficiency and a deep understanding of respiratory physiology. These procedures are not merely technical exercises; they are life-saving interventions that can mean the difference between life and death.

One specific scenario that sticks with me was a car accident where one of the victims suffered blunt force trauma to the chest, resulting in significant respiratory compromise. The rapid assessment indicated the need for advanced airway intervention, and the team was able to use rapid sequence intubation (RSI) to secure a definitive airway, saving the patient's life. The training in this procedure, honed through simulated and real-life experiences, had prepared us to deal with this extreme challenge. It was not a textbook scenario; it was a testament to the importance of thorough training and teamwork.

Beyond the individual skills, teamwork forms another vital pillar of paramedic practice. Effective communication, clear delegation, and mutual respect are crucial to efficient patient care, especially in the chaotic and often high-stakes environment of an emergency scene. The ability to work seamlessly with other emergency responders—firefighters, police officers, and hospital staff—requires not only competence but empathy, recognizing and respecting the roles and perspectives of every member of the team. This team-based dynamic is crucial for managing complex situations where efficient communication and clear delegation of tasks are essential.

Moreover, the mental and emotional demands of the job are often overlooked. The constant exposure to trauma, suffering, and death takes a significant toll. Developing coping mechanisms, seeking support from colleagues and supervisors, and maintaining a healthy work-life balance are all crucial to long-term well-being and resilience. The ability to compartmentalize experiences, to process the emotional impact of traumatic events without letting them overwhelm, is as important as the technical skills themselves. This ability isn't just about personal health;

it's about protecting the effectiveness of the team and preserving one's ability to provide quality patient care.

Finally, continuous learning and professional development are an ongoing commitment for paramedics. The field of emergency medicine is constantly evolving, with new research, new techniques, and new medications constantly emerging. Keeping abreast of the latest advancements, attending continuing education courses, and participating in professional development opportunities are crucial for maintaining competence and providing the highest quality of care. This commitment to lifelong learning is not a choice; it is a professional imperative that ensures not only the paramedic's own development but also the safety and well-being of the patients entrusted to their care.

The anatomy of a paramedic is not simply a list of skills and knowledge; it is a complex interplay of scientific understanding, practical proficiency, emotional resilience, and unwavering dedication to service. It is a journey of constant learning, adapting, and refining, fueled by the unwavering commitment to providing the best possible care to those in their most vulnerable moments. The sirens' call is answered not just with courage and idealism but with a profound understanding of the human body, the complexities of trauma, and the unwavering commitment to the ethical principles that guide the profession. It is a journey that demands both technical mastery and an unyielding dedication to compassion, resilience and professional integrity.

The sterile environment of the training facility, with its meticulously arranged mannequins and predictable scenarios, offered little preparation for the chaotic reality of my first real emergency call. The controlled chaos of simulations paled in comparison to the raw, unpredictable energy that surged through me as the dispatcher's voice crackled over the radio, the familiar cadence of the siren's wail suddenly amplifying the weight of responsibility. It wasn't the textbook scenario we'd rehearsed countless times; this was life or death, unfolding in real time, with the stakes impossibly high.

The address was a nondescript apartment complex on the city's outskirts, the kind where flickering streetlights cast long, ominous shadows. As we pulled up, the scene was a cacophony of flashing lights and agitated voices. A young woman, her face pale and etched with fear, wrung her hands as she pointed towards the building's entrance. Her brother, she explained, had collapsed while cooking dinner. The air hung heavy with the metallic tang of blood, a visceral reminder of the potential severity of the situation.

My partner, a seasoned veteran with a reassuring calm that I desperately sought to emulate, took charge. His movements were fluid, efficient, the product of years spent navigating similar crises. The systematic approach, ingrained during training, kicked in, albeit with a tremor of apprehension in my hands. Assessing the scene, identifying immediate threats, initiating care – each action felt magnified, scrutinized not just by my partner but by the silent judgment of the situation itself.

The apartment was small, cluttered, the air thick with the scent of burnt food. The young man lay on the floor, unconscious, a pool of blood spreading ominously beneath his head. It was a stark contrast to the pristine, antiseptic environment of the training lab. This wasn't a simulated injury; this was a real person, a life hanging in the balance.

The initial assessment was a blur of rapid actions: checking for responsiveness, assessing airway, breathing, and circulation, feeling for a pulse, listening for breath sounds. My heart pounded against my ribs, the adrenaline a potent cocktail of fear and focus. The seemingly simple tasks – palpation, auscultation – felt monumental, each action weighed with the understanding that a wrong move, a misjudgment, could have devastating consequences. The theoretical knowledge, painstakingly acquired through months of study, now had to translate into decisive action under intense pressure.

My hands trembled as I attempted to insert an IV line, my nervousness momentarily disrupting my concentration. I'd practiced the procedure countless times, yet the pressure of the real-world situation amplified the inherent difficulty. My partner, sensing my distress, offered a quiet word of encouragement, a subtle adjustment of my technique that instantly restored my confidence. It wasn't just a technical skill; it was an act of trust, a shared responsibility that anchored me to the present moment.

The patient's condition was serious. He was hypotensive, tachycardiac, showing signs of internal bleeding. Each action was deliberate, calculated, and coordinated with my partner. The weight of the situation, the knowledge that we were the only barrier between this young man and a potential fatal outcome, pressed down on us. We worked as a unit, our communication seamless, our actions synchronized, the product of rigorous training and the instinctive bond forged through shared experience. It wasn't just a medical emergency; it was a test of our abilities, our teamwork, our resilience.

The ambulance ride to the hospital was a blur of activity: monitoring vital signs, administering fluids and medications, ensuring the patient's airway remained open. The siren's wail, a constant companion, seemed to amplify the intensity of the moment. The quiet hum of the engine provided a contrast to the chaos of the scene we left behind, allowing a space for reflection, for a brief respite from the intensity of the emergency. Reaching the emergency room, the transfer of the patient was efficient and organized. The handover to the hospital staff – a concise, detailed report – marked the end of our immediate responsibility.

But the experience itself lingered, etched into my memory with an intensity that no simulation could ever replicate.

The days and weeks following this first real call were a whirlwind of emotions. The initial adrenaline rush gave way to introspection, a critical self-assessment of my performance. The relentless questioning – could I have done better? What could I have improved upon? – haunted me. The idealized view of the profession, fueled by television dramas and personal aspirations, was replaced by a deeper understanding of the true demands of paramedicine. This was not just about the adrenaline rush; it was about navigating the complexities of human suffering, managing intense emotional pressure, and confronting the mortality that permeated the job.

This wasn't an isolated incident. Each subsequent call brought its own unique challenges, its own set of variables, its own potential for both success and failure. A child with a seizure, a senior citizen with a heart attack, a motor vehicle accident involving multiple casualties – each scenario pushed my skills and resilience to their limits. The knowledge acquired through training provided a framework, a foundation upon which I could build, but it was the experience, the countless hours spent facing real-world challenges, that truly shaped me into a paramedic.

One particularly memorable call involved a late-night response to a suspected overdose. The scene was grim, the apartment bathed in the eerie glow of a flickering streetlamp. The victim, a young man, lay unconscious, his breathing shallow and labored. The scene itself exuded despair, underscoring the harsh realities of addiction and the devastating impact on families and communities. The textbook protocols took precedence, of course, but this wasn't just a physiological challenge; it was a human tragedy, a reminder of the complexities and vulnerabilities inherent in the human condition.

Yet, amidst the challenges, there were moments of profound reward. The gratitude in the eyes of a patient who had been pulled back from the brink of death, the relief on the faces of their loved ones, the quiet satisfaction of knowing that our intervention had made a tangible difference; these moments fueled the commitment, mitigating the inevitable burnout and emotional toll.

The transition from the training environment to the real world of emergency response is a crucible. It's a baptism by fire, a jarring shift from the predictability of simulations to the unpredictable reality of life-or-death scenarios. New paramedics often grapple with intense anxiety, self-doubt, and the overwhelming weight of responsibility. The fear of making a mistake, of misjudging a situation, is palpable, often leading to self-criticism and a sense of inadequacy.

Overcoming this is a process of self-discovery, one that requires self-awareness, a willingness to learn from mistakes, and the courage to seek support from colleagues and mentors. It's about building confidence through experience, learning to manage the emotional impact of traumatic events, and developing coping mechanisms that can endure the demands of the job.

The siren's call, initially answered with naive idealism, transforms into a complex symphony of emotions and experiences. It is a journey marked by challenges, self-doubt, and the constant pressure to perform at one's peak; yet, it is also a journey of profound reward, driven by the human need to alleviate suffering, to make a difference, to save lives. It's a privilege, and a responsibility we hold dearly. And it's a journey that only begins with that first call, a journey that shapes us, tests us, and ultimately, defines us.

The transition from student to practicing paramedic is jarring, a stark leap from the controlled environment of the training facility to the unpredictable chaos of real-world emergencies. While the theoretical knowledge and practiced skills are undeniably crucial, they form only a fraction of the foundation needed to thrive in this demanding profession. What truly sustains us, what allows us to navigate the emotional and physical toll, is the strength of our teamwork and the wisdom imparted through mentorship.

My first partner, a man named Mark, embodied this ideal. He wasn't just a skilled paramedic; he was a teacher, a guide, a calm presence in the maelstrom of emergencies. His experience wasn't just about mastering procedures; it was about understanding the human element, the subtle cues, the unspoken anxieties that often accompanied the physical symptoms. He taught me more than IV insertion and airway management; he taught me to read a scene, to anticipate needs, to communicate effectively not only with my partner but with patients and their families, often in highly charged emotional situations.

He had a knack for defusing tension with a well-placed joke or a quiet word of encouragement. I remember one particular call where we responded to a young woman suffering a severe panic attack. The apartment was small, cluttered, the air thick with the smell of stale cigarette smoke and fear. The woman was hyperventilating, her breaths shallow and rapid, her body trembling uncontrollably. Many new paramedics would have focused solely on the physiological aspects: oxygen administration, perhaps some medication. Mark, however, took a different approach. He knelt beside her, spoke softly, his tone calm and reassuring. He listened patiently as she described her anxieties, offering words of comfort and empathy rather than simply medical interventions. He spoke to her fear, not just her symptoms. It was a masterclass in compassionate care, something I've carried with me throughout my career.

The combination of skillful medical intervention and empathetic human connection ultimately stabilized her condition. This wasn't just about medical proficiency; it was about building trust, creating a space where she felt safe and understood. This experience underscored a crucial lesson: paramedicine isn't solely about treating physiological issues; it's fundamentally about navigating human interactions, understanding the emotional landscape surrounding the medical emergency. Mark's mentorship extended beyond the immediate confines of the ambulance. He took the time to debrief after each challenging call, allowing me to process the emotions, reflect on my performance, and learn from any mistakes. He fostered a culture of open communication, where asking questions wasn't seen as a sign of weakness but rather a critical step toward growth.

Mentorship, however, isn't always a formal process. It often arises organically, from the shared experiences and unspoken understanding between colleagues. I recall one instance where a particularly difficult cardiac arrest had left me feeling depleted and uncertain. I was doubting my abilities, second-guessing every decision made during the resuscitation. It was late; the silence in the ambulance bay offered little comfort. Sarah, a fellow paramedic known for her quiet competence and unwavering composure, simply walked up, offered me a cup of coffee, and listened patiently as I poured out my anxieties. She didn't offer unsolicited advice or judgment; she simply provided a safe space for me to vent, validating my feelings and reminding me that even the most experienced paramedics have moments of doubt. Her empathetic listening was, in itself, a powerful form of mentorship.

Effective teamwork extends beyond the immediate response. It involves a seamless exchange of information, clear communication, and a shared commitment to patient care. This isn't always easy. Personality clashes, differing approaches to patient management, and the inevitable stress of the job can create friction. Building strong teams requires a conscious effort to cultivate mutual respect, open communication, and a shared understanding of roles and responsibilities. I've witnessed teams where a lack of effective communication led to delays in treatment, misinterpretations of crucial information, and even near-misses. In contrast, I've also seen teams where the synergy was palpable, where each member instinctively knew their role, anticipated the needs of others, and worked together seamlessly to achieve the best possible out-come for the patient.

The differences are often subtle but significant. In a high-performing team, communication flows effortlessly. Information is exchanged concisely and accurately, leaving no room for misunderstanding. Members support each other, offering help and encouragement without hesitation. They acknowledge each other's strengths and weaknesses, utilizing each member's skills effectively. They approach challenges collaboratively, pooling their knowledge and expertise to find the best solutions. Such synergy was particularly evident in one call where we responded to a multiple-vehicle accident on a busy highway. The scene was chaotic: twisted metal, broken glass, and a chorus of moans and screams. The initial assessment was swift and efficient, each team member taking responsibility for a specific task, their actions coordinated to ensure no detail was overlooked. Our communication was fluid and precise, the verbal report to the hospital clear and complete. The efficient triage and organized transport of the injured underscored the importance of team-work and preparation.

Beyond the immediate response, however, is the ongoing effort to maintain team cohesion. Regular training sessions, both technical and interpersonal, are essential to sharpen skills and maintain a shared understanding of protocols. Team-building exercises can foster camaraderie and communication. Open and honest feedback, focused on improvement rather than criticism, creates a culture of continuous growth. Regular debriefs after challenging calls are not only crucial for processing trauma but also serve as opportunities to analyze performance, identify areas for improvement, and reinforce team bonds.

This is not simply about camaraderie; it is about resilience. The para-medic profession presents an onslaught of emotional and psychological stressors. The cumulative effect of witnessing trauma, managing critical situations, and confronting the fragility of life can be profound. Team support becomes a lifeline, a source of strength and resilience, enabling us to process the emotional toll and navigate the challenges without succumbing to burnout.

The value of mentorship extends far beyond initial training. Throughout my career, I have continued to learn from senior paramedics, observing their techniques, seeking their advice, and benefiting from their experience. The paramedic profession is a constant learning process; each call presents an opportunity to learn and grow. The wisdom gained through mentoring helps us navigate the complexities of the job, develop effective coping mechanisms, and maintain a commitment to our profession.

The siren's call is initially answered with idealism, but it's the ongoing support and guidance of our colleagues and mentors that provide the enduring strength and resilience needed to navigate this demanding profession. It is a testament to the power of teamwork, mentorship and camaraderie in shaping individuals into not just skilled paramedics, but compassionate professionals dedicated to serving our communities through the most challenging of circumstances. The journey is not only arduous; it is profoundly rewarding, filled with moments of immense satisfaction and a palpable sense of purpose. And it's a journey best traveled not alone, but alongside a supportive team and wise mentors.

The initial allure of paramedicine is potent; a siren song weaving tales of heroism, adrenaline-fueled rescues, and the profound satisfaction of making a tangible difference in people's lives. This idealistic vision, often nurtured during training, is a powerful motivator, drawing individuals to a career that demands immense skill, resilience, and compassion. However, the stark reality of the profession can be a jarring contrast to these romanticized notions. The transition from the structured, controlled environment of paramedic school to the chaotic unpredictability of real-world emergencies is a significant hurdle. It's a crucible that tests not only our technical abilities but also our emotional fortitude and psychological resilience.

One of the most significant adjustments is learning to manage expectations. The textbook scenarios we practiced during training rarely mirror the messy, complex reality of responding to an emergency. In school, patients often presented with textbook symptoms, allowing for a clear diagnosis and straightforward treatment. Real-life emergencies, however, are often far more ambiguous. Patients may be reluctant to share information, symptoms may be atypical or masked by other conditions, and the environment itself can be fraught with challenges—limited access, hostile bystanders, or scenes of intense emotional distress. This inherent unpredictability requires a level of adaptability and problem-solving that cannot be fully replicated in a classroom setting.

During my early years, I vividly remember the crushing weight of expectation. Every call felt like a high-stakes examination, my performance intensely scrutinized, both by myself and, implicitly, by my partner. The pressure to diagnose accurately, administer the correct treatment, and make life-or-death decisions was immense. The adrenaline rush, initially exhilarating, could quickly morph into crippling anxiety, leaving me feeling exhausted and emotionally drained. I recall one particular call where we responded to a man experiencing chest pain. While his symptoms pointed towards a heart attack, there were inconsistencies in his presentation. He was unusually calm, and his ECG was equivocal. The uncertainty was agonizing; the fear of making a critical error was palpable. Ultimately, his symptoms resolved themselves, but the lingering doubt gnawed at me for days. This wasn't simply a medical uncertainty; it was a profound test of my confidence and resilience.

Learning to navigate this uncertainty requires a fundamental shift in perspective. It's not about eliminating doubt entirely; it's about learning to manage it, to recognize it as a natural part of the process, and to develop strategies to cope with it. This begins with self-compassion. We must accept that mistakes are inevitable, that uncertainty is inherent in the profession, and that it is okay to question our decisions and seek support from our colleagues.

Another critical aspect of managing expectations is understanding the limitations of our role. We are not miracle workers; we cannot always save every patient, and some outcomes are simply beyond our control. This can be difficult to accept, especially when we've poured our hearts and souls into a resuscitation attempt only to witness a patient succumb to their injuries. The emotional toll of these experiences is immense, and learning to process these losses without allowing them to consume us is a vital skill. The notion of "saving lives" – a common motivator for entering the profession – needs to be nuanced. While saving lives remains a core aspect, it's equally important to accept that our role often involves mitigating suffering, providing comfort, and ensuring a dignified end of life. Sometimes, our greatest success is simply in offering compassion and support to patients and their families in their most vulnerable moments.

This acceptance is not a passive resignation but a conscious choice to redefine success. It is about recognizing the profound impact we can have, even in situations where a complete cure or reversal is impossible. It's about finding purpose in acts of comfort, in providing solace to grieving families, and in offering a sense of peace and dignity during a crisis.

M oreover, managing expectations involves recognizing the impact of the job on our own well-being. The cumulative effects of stress, trauma exposure, and emotional demands can take a significant toll on our mental and physical health. It's essential to establish healthy coping mechanisms, to prioritize self-care, and to seek support when needed. This may include mindfulness practices, regular exercise, healthy eating habits, and engaging in activities that promote relaxation and stress reduction. It also involves seeking professional help when necessary. There's no shame in seeking therapy or counseling; it's a sign of strength and self-awareness, not weakness. In fact, accessing mental health re-sources should be considered a crucial aspect of self-care, a proactive measure to protect both our well-being and our ability to serve our patients effectively.

The reality of paramedicine is a far cry from the idealized portrayals often seen in movies and television. There are long shifts, challenging working conditions, and constant exposure to trauma and human suffering. There is immense responsibility, significant pressure, and the ongoing threat of physical harm. However, this demanding profession is also profoundly rewarding. The moments of connection with patients, the tangible impact we can have, and the camaraderie shared with colleagues are invaluable. The ability to navigate this complex landscape, to balance the idealism with the realities, to maintain compassion and empathy amid the chaos—this is the essence of becoming a truly effective paramedic.

It's about fostering a realistic understanding of what this profession entails, acknowledging the emotional and mental toll, and actively developing coping mechanisms. It's about creating support networks among colleagues and building a robust personal support system outside of work. It's about continuous self-reflection and a commitment to ongoing professional development. It's about recognizing that while the siren's call initially beckons us with a promise of heroism, the true fulfillment lies in navigating the complexities of this challenging yet rewarding career with grace, resilience, and unwavering dedication. The journey is not one of unwavering heroism; it's a journey of ongoing adaptation, learning, and growth, a testament to the human spirit's capacity for empathy and resilience in the face of immense adversity. The challenge, therefore, is not in rejecting the idealism, but in refining it, in shaping it into a realistic, sustainable, and fulfilling career path. The initial idealism provides the fuel; the adaptability and self-awareness provide the navigation system to safely reach the destination.

2

In the Field: High-Pressure Situations and Ethical

The high-pitched wail of the siren, the flashing lights cutting through the pre-dawn darkness – these are the familiar preludes to a trauma call, a stark reminder of the unpredictable nature of our profession. While every call presents its own unique challenges, trauma calls occupy a special, often brutal, category. They are not merely emergencies; they are visceral encounters with human vulnerability, fragility, and often, profound loss. The physical demands are immense, the emotional toll even greater.

My first truly impactful trauma call involved a motorcycle accident. The scene was chaotic: twisted metal, shattered glass, the pungent smell of gasoline mingling with the metallic tang of blood. The victim, a young man, lay amidst the wreckage, his body contorted at an unnatural angle. The visual impact was jarring, a stark contrast to the sterile environments of the training simulations. The adrenaline surged, a potent cocktail of fear and determination. My training kicked in; we swiftly assessed the situation, initiated advanced life support, and worked to stabilize him for transport. But even amidst the controlled chaos of our actions, the raw brutality of the scene lingered, a persistent undercurrent of anxiety.

The physical demands of such calls are undeniable. We lift, we carry, we wrestle with equipment, often in cramped, difficult spaces. The strain on our bodies is cumulative, leading to chronic back pain, repetitive strain injuries, and a host of other physical ailments. Years of hoisting patients, navigating uneven terrain, and working long shifts in uncomfortable positions takes its toll. I remember one particularly grueling night involving a multiple-vehicle pile-up. We worked for hours in freezing rain, battling the elements as much as the injuries. By the end of the shift, my muscles ached, my body screamed for rest, yet the exhaustion was far surpassed by the emotional weight of the night's events.

But the physical challenges pale in comparison to the emotional aftermath. Trauma calls are intensely visceral experiences. We witness the raw, unfiltered consequences of human fallibility, the sudden and brutal disruption of life. We see the fear in a child's eyes, the resignation in the gaze of a dying man, the silent grief etched onto the faces of grieving family members. These images, these sounds, these smells – they become deeply etched into our memories. They replay themselves in our minds long after the shift ends, intruding upon our sleep, coloring our waking hours.

The emotional toll manifests in various ways. There's the immediate shock and adrenaline surge, followed by a period of intense focus and activity. But once the call is over, the adrenaline subsides, leaving behind a profound sense of exhaustion, a feeling of being emotionally drained. This can lead to irritability, difficulty sleeping, and an overall sense of being overwhelmed. In the long term, untreated trauma exposure can lead to Post-Traumatic Stress Disorder (PTSD), anxiety, depression, and burnout. We carry the weight of those experiences, the burden of witnessing human suffering, often in silence. The stories we don't tell, the silent screams we bear witness to, remain embedded in our subconscious, sometimes manifesting as nightmares, intrusive thoughts, or a pervasive sense of unease.

The challenge is to develop effective coping mechanisms to manage the emotional fallout of trauma calls. This begins with recognizing that our experiences are valid and that it's okay to feel overwhelmed, scared, or even angry. Denying these emotions only allows them to fester, potentially leading to more significant mental health issues. Self-compassion is paramount. We need to allow ourselves to process our emotions, to acknowledge the impact of the job on our mental well-being. This might involve talking to a trusted colleague, a family member, a therapist, or even journaling – finding an outlet to express the emotions that are often suppressed.

Peer support is crucial. Sharing experiences with colleagues who understand the unique challenges of paramedicine can be incredibly therapeutic. The ability to talk openly and honestly about the difficult calls, to know that you are not alone in your struggles, can provide a profound sense of relief and validation. Our professional culture, however, often discourages the open discussion of emotional distress, perpetuating a culture of silence that isolates and harms those who need support the most. We need to actively cultivate an environment where open communication and mutual support are valued and encouraged.

Beyond peer support, accessing professional mental health resources is vital. Seeking therapy is not a sign of weakness but a proactive measure to protect our mental well-being. Therapy provides a safe space to process traumatic experiences, develop coping mechanisms, and build resilience. Regular mindfulness practices, such as meditation or deep breathing exercises, can help to manage stress and regulate emotions. Engaging in activities that promote relaxation and self-care – spending time in nature, pursuing hobbies, connecting with loved ones – are crucial for maintaining a healthy work-life balance.

The challenge extends beyond individual coping mechanisms. Our organizational structures and training programs need to prioritize the mental health of paramedics. This includes providing readily accessible mental health resources, integrating mental health education into our training programs, and fostering a culture of support and understanding. Leaders in the field must actively address the stigma associated with seeking mental health care, encouraging open communication about emotional well-being, and fostering a culture of compassion and understanding.

The work we do is profoundly meaningful, yet it also comes with an immense emotional price. Learning to manage the physical and emotional toll of trauma calls is not a matter of individual resilience alone; it is a collective responsibility. It demands a comprehensive approach, encompassing individual self-care, peer support, access to mental health resources, and a fundamental shift in organizational culture. Only by recognizing and addressing this crucial aspect of paramedicine can we ensure the long-term well-being of our professionals and sustain the quality of care we provide to our communities. The siren's song may initially lure us with a promise of heroism, but the true measure of our success lies in our ability to navigate this demanding profession with both physical and emotional resilience, carrying with us not just the weight of our equipment but also the weight of our experiences with compassion, grace, and the unwavering support of our colleagues and community.

The emotional toll of trauma calls, as profoundly impactful as it is, represents only one facet of the challenges we face. Another, equally significant, layer is the ethical dimension – the constant barrage of difficult decisions made under immense pressure, often with life-or-death consequences. These aren't academic exercises; they are real-time moral dilemmas played out against the backdrop of sirens, flashing lights, and the desperate cries for help.

One recurring ethical challenge is resource allocation, particularly during mass casualty incidents (MCIs). The chilling reality of an MCI is the stark imbalance between the overwhelming need and the limited resources available. We are forced to make agonizing choices, prioritizing patients based on the likelihood of survival, a brutal calculus that often clashes with our innate desire to save everyone. I recall a horrific pile-up on a busy highway; dozens of injured, some critically so. The sheer number of victims, the cries for help, the sea of red and blue lights – it was a scene of unimaginable chaos. Our team, along with other emergency responders, were rapidly overwhelmed. We had to triage patients, assigning priorities based on a system that felt both necessary and profoundly unfair. Making those decisions, choosing who receives immediate care and who might have to wait, is a burden that weighs heavily long after the scene is cleared. It's a burden shared, but never fully relinquished. The image of a young mother, her face contorted in pain, while we worked on a more severely injured child, remains a haunting reminder of the agonizing choices we're sometimes forced to make.

The concept of "doing the most good for the most people" is deceptively simple in theory; it becomes a profoundly complex ethical quagmire in practice. What constitutes "most good"? Is it saving the most lives, or is there a moral imperative to prioritize those with the highest potential for a full recovery? And what about the ethical implications of making such choices under pressure, without the benefit of careful deliberation or consultation? There's no easy answer, no comforting algorithm to guide us through this moral thicket. We rely on training, experience, and a strong ethical compass, yet doubt lingers. We're left grappling with the implications of our actions long after we've left the scene.

End-of-life decisions present another critical ethical challenge. We are often the first responders to witness the final moments of a person's life. Sometimes, the decision to initiate or withhold life-sustaining treatment rests on our shoulders. This is particularly challenging when dealing with patients who lack decision-making capacity or have conflicting family wishes. We're forced to balance the medical imperative to preserve life with the patient's wishes, as best as we can ascertain them, and the ethical considerations surrounding quality of life. The weight of that responsibility can be immense, demanding not just medical expertise, but also profound empathy and a keen awareness of the ethical implications of our actions. One case stands out: an elderly patient, already frail and suffering, experiencing a catastrophic stroke. The family was deeply divided; some wanted to initiate aggressive life support, others wanted to allow nature to take its course. As paramedics, we had to carefully navigate the family's conflicting wishes, explain the implications of our actions, and ultimately support a decision that may have felt incomplete, yet was based on the best available information and ethical considerations. The emotional aftermath of such calls lingers, prompting self-reflection and professional growth.

The ethical complexities extend beyond these specific scenarios. We constantly grapple with issues of patient confidentiality, informed consent, and the boundaries of our scope of practice. Every decision, every action, has an ethical dimension. Maintaining patient confidentiality, even in high-stress situations, is not just a matter of following regulations; it is a fundamental aspect of professional integrity. Ensuring informed consent, however, can be fraught with challenges when dealing with patients in crisis, with impaired cognitive abilities, or in situations where information is limited or time is critical. This often involves balancing the need for urgent medical intervention with the patient's right to make autonomous decisions, a delicate dance between urgency and respect.

The pressure of these ethical dilemmas is amplified by the inherent limitations of the paramedic profession. We operate in unpredictable environments, with limited information, often under extremely stressful conditions. We make decisions on the fly, sometimes with incomplete data, relying on our training, experience, and our own sense of judgment. This adds a significant layer of complexity to the ethical considerations, making it all the more crucial to develop robust ethical reasoning skills. Training programs must incorporate scenarios and ethical dilemmas within the context of real-world pressure, preparing us to face the ethical challenges of the profession effectively.

Moreover, the lack of immediate oversight can intensify the ethical pressure. While we are bound by professional codes of conduct and legal frameworks, the immediate decision-making frequently falls solely on us. This autonomy can be both empowering and isolating, creating a situation where the burden of ethical judgment rests entirely on our shoulders. Post-incident reviews and debriefings are essential, but they rarely mitigate the immediate emotional impact of grappling with these complex ethical dilemmas in real-time.

The lack of readily available ethical support or supervision further complicates the matter. Paramedics need readily accessible guidance and consultation. The creation of ethics committees within EMS organizations, the development of accessible hotlines for immediate advice, and regular ethics training could help mitigate some of the ethical burdens. A supportive, non-judgmental environment within EMS organizations, where open discussion of ethical dilemmas is encouraged, would foster an atmosphere of mutual learning and support. This would foster a culture where mistakes aren't viewed as failures, but rather as opportunities for learning and growth. This would, ultimately, improve the quality of ethical decision-making and better protect the well-being of paramedics.

Reflecting on my experiences, I believe that developing robust ethical reasoning skills is not merely a matter of memorizing codes of conduct. It is a process of continuous learning, critical reflection, and a commitment to ethical awareness. We must engage in ongoing education, participating in ethics workshops, reflecting on our experiences, and seeking guidance from mentors and peers. Developing a personal ethical framework, grounded in our own values and professional principles, is essential. This isn't a passive process; it requires continuous effort, introspection, and a commitment to aligning our actions with our ethical principles. There's no room for complacency; the ethical challenges of paramedicine demand constant attention, self-reflection and a willingness to learn and adapt.

The ethical dimension of paramedicine is profoundly complex and deeply intertwined with the emotional and physical realities of the job. It's a constant negotiation between our training, experience, and personal values, played out against the backdrop of life-or-death situations. Recognizing this complexity, embracing the moral challenges, and fostering a culture of ethical reflection and support are not merely professional obligations; they are crucial for the well-being of paramedics and the quality of care we provide. The siren's wail is a summons to action, but it's also a call for reflection, demanding that we examine our actions, learn from our experiences, and strive to provide the best possible care, both ethically and medically.

The ethical considerations we've explored are inextricably linked to the critical thinking skills required in the field. Every decision, from initiating CPR to administering medication, hinges on rapid assessment and the application of our knowledge and experience. This is where the rubber truly meets the road, the theoretical knowledge gained in training transformed into life-saving action under immense pressure. It's a high-stakes game of medical chess, where every move carries profound consequences.

One of the most critical skills is the ability to quickly assess a patient's condition. This is not simply a checklist of vital signs; it's a holistic evaluation, taking into account the patient's presentation, the circumstances surrounding the incident, and the available information. A seemingly simple fall, for instance, could mask a more serious underlying condition like a stroke or a heart attack. Our training equips us to recognize subtle signs and symptoms, to discern patterns that point towards a diagnosis, even in the midst of chaos. The ability to quickly distinguish between a minor injury and a life-threatening emergency is paramount, dictating our priority and influencing subsequent treatment decisions. It's a skill honed through years of experience and constant learning, a sixth sense developed through countless encounters with the spectrum of human suffering.

Intuition plays a surprising, yet critical, role in this rapid assessment process. It's that gut feeling, that almost inexplicable sense that something isn't quite right, even when the objective data might not fully support it. It's a combination of experience, pattern recognition, and an almost preternatural awareness of the subtle nuances of human physiology. I remember a case where an elderly woman presented with what appeared to be a simple case of dehydration. Her vital signs were stable, and she was alert and oriented. Yet, something felt off. My intuition told me to delve deeper. A thorough secondary assessment revealed a subtle irregularity in her heart rhythm, which later confirmed a cardiac issue requiring immediate intervention. Without that intuitive nudge, a critical diagnosis might have been missed.

While intuition provides a crucial initial assessment, it must be rigorously validated by objective data. We don't simply rely on gut feelings; we meticulously gather information through physical examination, patient history, and the use of diagnostic tools. The systematic approach honed during training, often using mnemonic devices like SAMPLE (Symptoms, Allergies, Medications, Past Medical History, Last Oral Intake, Events leading to the illness/injury) provides the structured framework within which our intuition can operate. It is a constant interplay between objective data and subjective interpretation, a delicate balancing act between scientific rigor and experiential insight.

Rapid treatment is often as crucial as rapid assessment. We don't have the luxury of lengthy deliberations; every second counts. This requires a deep understanding of pharmacology, procedural skills, and the ability to adapt to rapidly changing situations. We are essentially practicing medicine in a moving emergency room, with limited resources and ever-evolving circumstances. A strong grasp of basic life support, advanced cardiac life support, and trauma management is non-negotiable. But beyond the technical proficiency, it's the ability to apply these skills creatively and effectively under pressure that truly distinguishes a skilled paramedic.

One particularly challenging aspect is managing uncertainty. We often operate with incomplete information, faced with ambiguous presentations and rapidly evolving situations. This requires a flexible and adaptable approach, the ability to adjust treatment plans based on new information and changing circumstances. It's about accepting that we won't always have all the answers, and that making decisions with incomplete information is part and parcel of the job. This often involves making educated guesses, weighing the potential risks and benefits of various interventions, and trusting our judgment.

The ability to collaborate effectively is equally vital. Paramedicine is a team sport. Effective communication, efficient teamwork, and mutual respect are essential for navigating the complex dynamics of emergency response. This involves clear and concise communication with the patient, family members, other first responders, and hospital staff. It also requires the ability to delegate tasks effectively, manage team dynamics, and maintain composure under pressure.

Beyond the immediate technical skills, critical thinking in the field demands a profound level of emotional intelligence. We are constantly dealing with people at their most vulnerable, confronting their fears,

anxieties, and often, profound grief. The ability to connect with patients on a human level, to provide comfort and reassurance amidst the
chaos, is as crucial as any medical intervention. This empathy allows us
to build trust, obtain essential information, and administer care in a way
that is both effective and compassionate. It's a delicate balance between
maintaining professional boundaries and showing genuine human connection.

Continuous learning is another cornerstone of critical thinking in
the field. The field of medicine, and especially emergency medical services, is constantly evolving. New research, advances in technology, and
updated guidelines require constant updating of our knowledge and
skills. This necessitates a commitment to lifelong learning, a willingness
to embrace new information and to adapt our practice accordingly.
Keeping abreast of the latest evidence-based practices is not just a professional obligation; it's a matter of patient safety.

Finally, and perhaps most importantly, critical thinking in the field
necessitates a healthy dose of self-reflection. We must be willing to critically evaluate our own performance, identify our weaknesses, and learn
from our mistakes. This process of self-assessment is crucial for professional growth, and it's a cornerstone of continuous improvement.
Post-incident reviews and debriefings offer invaluable opportunities for
self-reflection, fostering a culture of learning and improvement within
our teams.

In the crucible of a high-pressure emergency, critical thinking is not
just a desirable skill; it is the foundation upon which our ability to provide effective and ethical care rests. It is a tapestry woven from clinical
knowledge, technical proficiency, experiential insight, emotional intelligence, collaborative teamwork, continuous learning, and unwavering
self-reflection. It's a skill that is honed over time, tested in the fires of
crisis, and refined through the constant process of learning and adapta-

tion. This isn't just about treating the injuries; it is about understanding the whole person, the context of their situation, and the ethical implications of each decision. It is this multifaceted, holistic approach that defines truly effective paramedicine.

The adrenaline surge, the chaotic scene, the myriad of flashing lights – these are the hallmarks of an emergency response. But amidst the frenzy, effective communication is the bedrock upon which successful interventions are built. It's not just about shouting orders; it's about conveying crucial information accurately, calmly, and efficiently to a diverse range of individuals under immense pressure. This involves not only verbal communication but also non-verbal cues, active listening, and a keen awareness of the emotional states of those involved.

I vividly recall a particularly chaotic night involving a multi-vehicle pile-up on a rain-slicked highway. The scene was a cacophony of sirens, twisted metal, and anguished cries. Multiple patients, each with varying degrees of injury, needed immediate attention. My partner and I, working in tandem with the fire department and police, had to coordinate our efforts seamlessly. The initial minutes were crucial, demanding precise communication to establish a clear chain of command, assign roles, and prioritize patients based on their criticality. Shouting orders wouldn't work; the noise level was too high. Instead, we utilized hand signals, pre-established codes, and short, crisp radio transmissions, conveying vital information without adding to the noise. This pre-planned communication strategy, developed during training, became our lifeline in that maelstrom of activity. It allowed us to maintain order and ensure the most critically injured patients received immediate care while other teams assessed less severely injured victims.

Effective communication isn't just about efficiency; it's also about building rapport and trust, particularly with frightened and injured patients. In the midst of pain and fear, a patient needs to feel understood and reassured. A calm, empathetic voice, a gentle touch, and clear explanations can go a long way in reducing anxiety and facilitating a more effective assessment. I often find myself employing active listening techniques—repeating back key information the patient provides, asking clarifying questions, and validating their feelings—to foster a sense of trust and cooperation. This approach helps not only in gathering crucial medical history but also in providing emotional support during a vulnerable time. The simple act of making eye contact, offering a reassuring smile, or gently holding a patient's hand can sometimes be as effective as any medication.

Communication extends beyond the patient. Clear, concise communication with bystanders is equally essential. An uncontrolled crowd can easily become a significant hazard at an emergency scene. Providing clear and concise instructions, keeping bystanders at a safe distance, and reassuring them about the actions being taken can help prevent further complications. In certain situations, a bystander may possess critical information about the event that could impact patient care. A well-placed question, delivered with empathy, can unlock essential details that may not otherwise be apparent.

Collaborating with other first responders, such as fire and police personnel, is paramount. Emergency medical services are a collaborative effort, demanding a seamless integration of skills and expertise. This requires a shared understanding of roles and responsibilities, established protocols, and a common language. Consistent use of radio codes and standard operating procedures ensures clear and unambiguous communication, minimizing potential misunderstandings in high-pressure situations. I've found that fostering a respectful and collaborative relationship with other responders is essential for successful teamwork. It's through regular joint training exercises and informal interactions that we build trust and develop a shared understanding of each other's capabilities.

Furthermore, seamless communication with hospital staff is crucial for ensuring a smooth handover of care. Providing a comprehensive report, including the patient's vital signs, medical history, treatment given, and any ongoing concerns, is critical for facilitating continuous care in the hospital environment. A clear, well-organized handover report saves valuable time and ensures that the receiving medical team has all the information needed to provide timely and effective treatment. The efficient exchange of information minimizes potential errors and contributes to the overall safety and well-being of the patient. This collaborative approach extends beyond the immediate emergency response; it represents a continuous chain of care aimed at providing the best possible outcomes for our patients.

Beyond the technical aspects, effective communication relies heavily on emotional intelligence. Paramedics are often the first to encounter trauma, both physical and emotional. We witness accidents, injuries, and even death, situations that can be deeply disturbing, not only for the patient and their families, but also for ourselves. Therefore, emotional resilience is key. This necessitates not only understanding our own emotional responses but also recognizing and responding to the emotional needs of those around us. This involves actively listening to concerns, validating emotions, and providing empathy and reassurance, even in the face of overwhelming demands. It's a skill honed over years of experience, often learned through both success and setbacks.

The ability to handle difficult conversations is also crucial. Delivering bad news, providing difficult diagnoses, or dealing with angry or distressed family members neessitates exceptional communication skills. Approaching these situations with empathy, patience, and sensitivity is vital for maintaining a professional, yet human, connection. I recall having to deliver the news of a fatality to a distraught family member. The words themselves are insignificant in the face of such devastating loss.

What made the difference was a quiet presence, a listening ear, and a genuine expression of empathy. It was a profoundly moving experience, underlining the imortance of compassionate communication in the face of tragic loss.

Effective communication and collaboration are not innate abilities; they are skills that are refined through continuous practice and learning. Participation in regular training sessions focused on communication techniques, scenario-based simulations, and post-incident debriefings are essential for improving both individual and team performance. These learning opportunities provide valuable feedback and allow for the identification of areas needing improvement, fostering a culture of continuous learning and refinement. Regular feedback from super-visors, peers, and even patients is invaluable in identifying strengths and weaknesses, contributing to overall professional development. This process of self-reflection and continuous improvement is paramount for maintaining a high standard of care and ensuring that our communica-tion remains effective and compassionate.

In the fast-paced and high-stakes environment of paramedicine, seamless communication and collaboration are not just desirable traits; they are the very pillars of effective care. They're the threads that weave together the disparate elements of an emergency response, transforming chaos into coordinated action, fear into reassurance, and ultimately, transforming a crisis into an opportunity for healing. It's a dance of words, actions, and empathy, a symphony of coordinated efforts that, when executed correctly, can make the difference between life and death. This understanding is not just theoretical; it's a lived experience, a con-stant lesson learned and relearned on every call, in every situation, every day. The ability to effectively communicate and collaborate, therefore, is not simply a skill—it is the defining characteristic of a truly exceptional paramedic.

The chaotic ballet of an emergency scene often feels less like a well-rehearsed performance and more like a constantly shifting improvisation. One moment, you're dealing with a straightforward laceration; the next, a cascading series of unforeseen complications throws your initial assessment into disarray. This inherent unpredictability is the defining characteristic of paramedicine, demanding a level of adaptability and problem-solving prowess rarely found outside of high-stakes environments. It's not simply about possessing the knowledge; it's about the ability to apply that knowledge creatively and decisively in the face of uncertainty.

I remember a call involving a hiker who had fallen down a steep embankment. Initially, the report suggested a sprained ankle. Upon arrival, however, the scene painted a far more complex picture. The patient was conscious but disoriented, complaining of severe back pain and exhibiting signs of internal bleeding. Accessing the patient was a challenge in itself, requiring a coordinated effort with the fire department's technical rescue team. The terrain was treacherous, the light fading fast, and the patient's condition rapidly deteriorating. Our initial plan—a straightforward extrication and transport—had to be scrapped entirely.

The uncertainty forced us to think on our feet. We needed to reassess the patient's condition, adapt our extrication strategy, and simultaneously manage a potential deterioration in his vital signs. We established a clear communication channel with the rescue team, adjusting our plan to accommodate the rugged terrain and the patient's precarious condition. This involved improvising a makeshift stretcher using readily available materials, modifying our radio communication protocol to handle the challenges of the terrain, and providing immediate, albeit limited, pain management due to the inaccessibility of more sophisticated techniques.

It wasn't just about the technical challenges; we also had to contend with the emotional toll of the situation. The patient, already in considerable pain, was becoming increasingly anxious as he became aware of the complexity of the rescue. Reassuring him while coordinating the efforts of the rescue team, managing his vital signs, and strategizing the best way to extricate him from the precarious situation required a delicate balance of decisive action and compassionate care. This necessitated not only the ability to adapt and problem-solve but also a significant dose of emotional intelligence.

Adaptability in paramedicine extends beyond the immediate scene. We often have to make crucial decisions with incomplete information, weighing the potential risks and benefits of different treatment options. For example, a patient presenting with chest pain could be suffering from anything from a simple case of indigestion to a life-threatening heart attack. Making the right call, quickly and accurately, requires a clinical judgment based on both experience and the ability to integrate seemingly disparate pieces of information. This involves not only recognizing the relevant symptoms but also understanding the context – the patient's medical history, lifestyle, and current circumstances.

In such situations, our training serves as a framework, but our experience shapes our decisions. We learn to identify patterns, recognize subtle clues, and anticipate potential complications. This isn't a purely intellectual process; it's deeply intertwined with our intuition, honed through years of exposure to a wide spectrum of medical emergencies. It's the cumulative effect of hundreds, if not thousands, of calls, each one adding to our experience base and refining our ability to navigate uncertainty.

Furthermore, our ability to solve problems in the field is often tested not only by medical challenges but also by logistical ones. Resource constraints, unpredictable weather conditions, or the sheer complexity of a multi-casualty incident can all add significant layers of difficulty. We learn to prioritize, to delegate tasks effectively, and to make the most of the resources available to us, often under tremendous time pressure.

I recall a particularly challenging winter night where a blizzard had crippled the roads, rendering many areas inaccessible. We received a call about a young child experiencing respiratory distress in a remote rural area. The route was perilous, the roads choked with snow and ice. Our initial plan – a straightforward drive to the scene – was immediately rendered unfeasible. We had to adapt our strategy, coordinating with the local fire department to use a snowmobile to reach the child, all while communicating with the dispatch center and the hospital to prepare for the child's arrival.

The decision-making process involved weighing the risks and benefits of different transport methods, considering the child's deteriorating condition against the dangers of navigating the treacherous roads. The situation demanded not only technical proficiency but also a cool head, the ability to make rapid but informed decisions under immense pressure, and a willingness to improvise and adapt to ever-changing circumstances.

Effective problem-solving in emergency medical situations goes beyond technical skills; it's fundamentally about critical thinking and clinical reasoning. It involves the ability to systematically analyze the situation, gather relevant information, generate potential solutions, and evaluate the pros and cons of each option before making a final decision. This cognitive process is significantly enhanced by experience, teamwork, and constant learning.

Regular training exercises, involving scenario-based simulations and post-incident analysis, are crucial for developing these skills. These exercises allow us to practice our problem-solving abilities in a safe environment, identifying our strengths and weaknesses, and refining our strategies for handling unforeseen complications. Furthermore, debriefings after high-pressure calls allow us to learn from our experiences, to analyze our decisions, and to improve our approach to future situations.

This iterative process of learning, refinement, and adaptation is paramount in a field where uncertainty is the constant. It's the cornerstone of effective paramedic practice, allowing us to navigate the complexities of emergency medicine, to meet the challenges of unpredictable situations, and ultimately, to deliver the best possible care to our patients, even when the path is anything but clear. The ability to adapt and solve problems, therefore, is not merely a skill; it's the very essence of what defines a truly capable paramedic. It's a testament to our resilience, our resourcefulness, and our unwavering commitment to providing life-saving care, even amidst the unknown.

3

Between Calls: The Impact on Mental Health

The relentless pace of paramedicine, the constant exposure to suffering, and the inherent emotional weight of life-and-death decisions can take a profound toll. While we are trained to handle the physical demands of the job, the emotional and psychological consequences often go unaddressed, leading to a condition known as compassion fatigue. It's not simply burnout; it's a deeper, more insidious erosion of empathy and resilience. It's the gradual dimming of the light that once fueled our passion for helping others.

I've seen it firsthand in colleagues, the subtle shift in demeanor, the weariness etched not just on their faces but in the depths of their eyes. It manifests in different ways, sometimes subtly, sometimes dramatically. One colleague, a veteran paramedic with years of experience, began exhibiting signs of detachment. The vibrant energy that once characterized him was replaced by a quiet resignation, a pervasive sense of emotional numbness. He'd always been the first to crack a joke, to offer a reassuring word to a distraught family member; now, he seemed distant, almost withdrawn. It was a heartbreaking transformation to witness.

Compassion fatigue isn't a sign of weakness; it's a testament to the intensity of the work we do. It's the cumulative effect of witnessing suffering, of confronting death, of bearing the weight of others' trauma. It's the price we pay for bearing witness to humanity's vulnerability, its fragility, and its capacity for both immense joy and profound sorrow.

The symptoms are often insidious, creeping in gradually until they become overwhelming. They can include emotional exhaustion, cynicism, depersonalization—a feeling of emotional detachment from patients and colleagues—and a reduced sense of personal accomplishment. You might find yourself increasingly irritable, struggling to maintain healthy relationships, or experiencing difficulty concentrating. Sleep disturbances, changes in appetite, and physical ailments are also common, a manifestation of the body's inability to cope with the relentless stress.

One of the most heartbreaking aspects of compassion fatigue is the erosion of empathy. This isn't a conscious choice; it's a self-protective mechanism, a way for the mind and body to cope with the sheer volume of emotional trauma. The constant exposure to suffering can lead to a sense of emotional overload, a need to distance oneself from the pain to avoid being overwhelmed. This emotional detachment, however, can lead to a sense of isolation, a feeling of being disconnected not only from patients but also from colleagues and loved ones.

The causes are multifaceted. The nature of our work is inherently stressful. We respond to emergencies, often involving traumatic injuries, sudden death, and the suffering of others. We witness violence, grief, and loss on a regular basis. The unpredictability of the job, the long hours, and the irregular work schedule add to the stress. Furthermore, the emotional burden of dealing with patients and their families, often in highly stressful situations, can be overwhelming. Add to this the administrative burdens, the paperwork, and the constant pressure to perform at the highest level, and you have a recipe for burnout and compassion fatigue.

I remember one particularly difficult call involving a young child who had been involved in a serious car accident. The scene was chaotic, the child's injuries severe. Despite our best efforts, the child succumbed to their injuries. The memory of the parents' raw grief, their inconsolable sorrow, stayed with me long after the call. That single call, while extreme, exemplifies the cumulative toll of constantly confronting such intense emotions. It's these experiences, amplified over time and compounded by other stressors, that contribute significantly to the development of compassion fatigue.

Another factor is the lack of adequate support systems. Often, paramedics work in isolation, with limited opportunities to debrief or process their experiences. The culture of stoicism, the unspoken expectation that we should be able to handle everything, can prevent us from seeking help when we need it most. We are trained to be strong, to be resilient, but this can inadvertently create a barrier to seeking support.

Recognizing the signs of compassion fatigue is the first step towards addressing it. It's crucial to be self-aware, to pay attention to our emotional and physical well-being. Regular self-reflection, journaling, and mindfulness practices can help us identify the subtle shifts in our emotions and behavior. Open communication with colleagues and supervisors is also essential. Creating a supportive work environment where it's acceptable to talk about the emotional challenges of the job is crucial for preventing compassion fatigue and promoting mental well-being.

Seeking professional help is not a sign of weakness; it's a sign of strength. Therapists specializing in trauma and first responders can provide valuable support, helping us process our experiences and develop coping strategies. Peer support groups, where paramedics can share their experiences and learn from each other, can also be invaluable. Remember, you are not alone in this. Many others have walked this path, and there is help available.

Prevention is key. Engaging in regular self-care practices is crucial. This includes getting enough sleep, eating a healthy diet, exercising regularly, and making time for activities that we find enjoyable and relaxing. Developing strong social connections, spending time with loved ones, and maintaining a healthy work-life balance are also essential. Learning to set boundaries, to say no when we need to, is vital in protecting our mental and emotional well-being.

The importance of debriefing after stressful calls cannot be overstated. These debriefings provide a safe space to process our emotions, to share our experiences, and to learn from each other. They allow us to normalize our feelings, to acknowledge the emotional toll of the job, and to develop effective coping strategies. Instituting regular debriefing sessions, whether formal or informal, is crucial in mitigating the risks of compassion fatigue.

Remember the human element in all this. Compassion fatigue isn't just about the numbers, the statistics, or the procedures; it's about the people we serve and the impact they have on us. The ability to connect with patients on a human level is essential to our work, but it also makes us vulnerable. It's this vulnerability, this capacity for empathy, that makes us great paramedics, but it's also what makes us susceptible to compassion fatigue. Protecting this empathy, cherishing this capacity for compassion, is crucial not only for our own well-being but also for the continued effectiveness of the care we provide. It requires ongoing vigilance, proactive self-care, and a willingness to seek help when we need it. Recognizing the signs, understanding the causes, and proactively engaging in self-care are essential steps in maintaining our mental and emotional well-being, ensuring that we can continue to provide the highest level of care while protecting ourselves from the insidious effects of compassion fatigue.

The relentless pressure cooker of paramedic work doesn't just affect us individually; it ripples outwards, impacting the most precious relationships in our lives. The emotional toll, the constant exposure to trauma, and the irregular hours can strain even the strongest bonds. It's a subtle erosion, often unnoticed until the cracks become fissures, threatening to shatter what we hold most dear. I've seen it countless times – the strained silences during family dinners, the missed birthdays, the growing distance between partners, the unspoken resentment simmering beneath the surface.

One of the most common challenges is the difficulty in explaining the job to those outside of it. How do you articulate the weight of carrying life-or-death responsibility, the emotional cost of witnessing unspeakable suffering, to someone who hasn't experienced it? It's like trying to describe the color blue to a person born blind; the understanding simply isn't there. The disconnect can lead to feelings of isolation, making it harder to share our experiences and receive the support we desperately need. My wife, bless her heart, has tried her best to understand, but there are moments – particularly after a particularly grueling shift involving a child – where the chasm between our worlds feels insurmountable. She can see the exhaustion, the emptiness in my eyes, but the sheer weight of what I carry remains invisible, unquantifiable. She asks how my day was, and I offer a vague, dismissive answer, terrified of unleashing the torrent of emotions held captive within.

The irregular hours are another significant hurdle. Working nights, weekends, and holidays means missing important events, family gatherings, and precious moments with loved ones. It leads to a sense of guilt and resentment, both within the relationship and within ourselves. We yearn to be present, to share in the joys and sorrows of our families, but the demands of the job often prevent us from doing so. I remember missing my daughter's first steps because I was attending to a critical patient. The memory still stings, a constant reminder of the sacrifices the job demands, a sacrifice that extends beyond our own personal well-being.

Then there's the emotional baggage we carry home. The stories of trauma, the raw grief witnessed, and the constant exposure to suffering can be difficult to leave at the station. The images and emotions cling to us, seeping into our personal lives, affecting our interactions with family and friends. The seemingly innocuous events – a car accident on the news, a child falling down – can trigger flashbacks and an overwhelming surge of emotions. This can be confusing and frustrating for our loved ones, leaving them feeling inadequate in their attempts to comfort or support us.

The solution isn't simply to "compartmentalize" our work and personal lives. That approach, while tempting, is ultimately unsustainable and detrimental to our mental health and relationships. Rather, we need to cultivate open and honest communication. It's about finding a way to express the emotional weight of the job without burdening our loved ones, without making them feel responsible for fixing something that is beyond their capacity to repair. This requires a conscious effort to find healthy ways to process our emotions, to debrief with trusted colleagues, or to seek professional help when needed.

One of the most effective strategies is to set clear boundaries. We need to learn to say no, to prioritize our well-being and the well-being of our relationships. This means consciously disconnecting from work during our time off, setting aside dedicated time for family and friends, and protecting our mental and emotional space. It means putting away the phone, resisting the urge to constantly check emails or news updates, and focusing on the present moment.

Prioritizing quality time together is crucial. It's not about the quantity of time spent but the quality of connection. Engaging in shared activities that foster intimacy and strengthen our bonds is essential. Even simple acts of kindness, like listening attentively, showing empathy, and expressing appreciation, can make a significant difference. It is important to actively work on fostering those connections, setting aside time specifically for these interactions. This might involve scheduling regular date nights, participating in family activities, or engaging in hobbies together. The key is to intentionally create moments of connection.

Seeking professional support shouldn't be viewed as a weakness but as a sign of strength. Therapy can provide a safe space to process our experiences, develop healthy coping mechanisms, and improve our communication skills. Couple's counseling can be particularly valuable in addressing relationship challenges stemming from the demands of the job. It is a place where you can openly discuss your experiences, and where your partner can process their own experiences and feelings regarding the impact of your job on your relationship. It allows for a deeper understanding and can help you develop strategies to navigate challenges more effectively.

Regular self-care is not a luxury; it is a necessity. Prioritizing physical health, through regular exercise, healthy eating, and sufficient sleep, will improve our overall well-being, making us better equipped to handle the stresses of our job and better partners and family members. Engaging in activities that bring us joy and relaxation is also crucial. These could be anything from reading to hiking, meditation to spending time in nature. The key is to find activities that help us de-stress, recharge, and reconnect with ourselves.

Finally, it is critical to cultivate empathy and understanding within our relationships. Our loved ones may not fully grasp the reality of our work, but by patiently educating them, we can foster a greater degree of understanding and compassion. It's not about expecting them to solve our problems but creating a space where we can share our experiences and receive support. It's about fostering mutual understanding and appreciation.

Maintaining healthy relationships as a paramedic requires conscious effort, commitment, and a willingness to seek help when needed. It's a continuous process, not a destination, demanding ongoing self-reflection, open communication, and a relentless pursuit of balance between the demands of the job and the needs of our personal lives. It's a journey of self-discovery, of learning to navigate the complexities of our profession while nurturing the most important relationships in our lives. The rewards, however, are immeasurable – the strength of bonds forged in the crucible of shared experiences, the unwavering love and support that sustains us through the darkest hours, and the enduring power of human connection in the face of immense adversity. This is the silent heroism often overlooked, the strength of a support system that holds us together, piece by piece, call by call.

The relentless demands of paramedic work extend far beyond the emergency scene. The emotional and physical toll accumulates, demanding a proactive and multifaceted approach to self-care. This isn't a luxury; it's a survival strategy, a cornerstone of our ability to continue serving our communities effectively and maintain healthy, fulfilling lives outside the ambulance. Neglecting our own well-being is a disservice not only to ourselves but also to our loved ones and the patients who depend on us.

Let's start with the foundation: physical health. This isn't about achieving some unrealistic fitness ideal, but about building a resilient body capable of withstanding the rigors of the job. Many of us lead sedentary lives between calls, sitting for extended periods in the ambulance or at the station. This lifestyle is a recipe for weight gain, muscle atrophy, and decreased cardiovascular fitness. The consequences extend beyond physical discomfort. Fatigue, low energy levels, and reduced physical stamina directly impact our ability to perform effectively during emergencies, increasing the risk of injury and burnout.

My own experience serves as a cautionary tale. During my early years, I prioritized work above all else, routinely sacrificing sleep and proper nutrition. The result was a vicious cycle of fatigue, poor decision-making, and increasing irritability. I vividly remember a particularly challenging night shift where I felt completely drained, both mentally and physically. It was a wake-up call. I recognized the urgent need for a fundamental shift in my approach to self-care.

The first step was incorporating regular physical activity into my routine. I started with small, achievable goals, such as a 30-minute walk most evenings. Gradually, I increased the intensity and duration of my workouts. Finding an exercise modality that I genuinely enjoyed was crucial. For me, it was running. The rhythmic pounding of my feet against the pavement became a form of meditation, a way to clear my head and process the stresses of the day. For others, it might be cycling, swimming, weightlifting, or any activity that promotes both cardiovascular health and strength training.

Along with regular exercise, I prioritized proper nutrition. This doesn't mean adhering to any restrictive diet; it's about making conscious choices that fuel my body with the nutrients it needs to function optimally. I began focusing on whole, unprocessed foods, limiting sugar and processed carbohydrates. Hydration became a priority, constantly replenishing fluids, especially after strenuous shifts. Learning to prepare healthy meals ahead of time became crucial, eliminating the temptation of grabbing quick, unhealthy options when time was short. This shift in dietary habits resulted in improved energy levels, better sleep, and a significant increase in overall well-being.

Sleep is often the first casualty of a demanding work schedule. Yet, it's arguably the most critical component of self-care. Sleep deprivation significantly impairs cognitive function, decision-making, and emotional regulation. It increases the risk of making errors in the field, putting both ourselves and our patients at risk. I experimented with various sleep hygiene techniques – establishing a regular sleep schedule, creating a relaxing bedtime routine, optimizing my sleep environment, and limiting screen time before bed. These changes gradually improved my sleep quality and reduced the persistent fatigue I had experienced. It is important to actively prioritize sleep, viewing it not as a luxury, but a fundamental requirement for physical and mental restoration.

Beyond the physical, mental well-being is equally, if not more, crucial. Paramedic work exposes us to constant stress, trauma, and moral dilemmas. The cumulative effect can lead to burnout, anxiety, depression, and even post-traumatic stress disorder (PTSD). Developing effective stress management techniques is therefore non-negotiable.

Mindfulness practices, such as meditation and deep breathing exercises, proved invaluable in managing stress and enhancing emotional regulation. Even a few minutes of daily mindfulness can have a profound impact, reducing anxiety and improving focus. I started by incorporating short guided meditation sessions into my daily routine, using apps specifically designed for stress reduction. The benefits quickly became apparent. I found myself better equipped to handle stressful situations, both in the field and in my personal life. These techniques are not merely about relaxation; they are about cultivating self-awareness and developing a healthier relationship with our thoughts and emotions.

Another powerful tool in my self-care arsenal is journaling. Writing down my thoughts and feelings allows me to process my experiences without judgment, to identify patterns of stress and develop strategies for managing them effectively. It's a form of emotional release, a space where I can explore my feelings without fear of reprisal or judgment. This process can help clarify and process emotions stemming from traumatic calls, assisting in the prevention of their further escalation.

Beyond these individual strategies, building a strong support system is paramount. This might involve connecting with colleagues, seeking professional counseling, or joining support groups specifically designed for paramedics. Sharing experiences with others who understand the unique challenges of the profession can provide a sense of validation, reducing feelings of isolation and fostering a sense of community. Moreover, having a trusted network to confide in during challenging times is critical. This support system shouldn't be considered a weakness but rather a critical element in managing the intense pressures of this career.

Seeking professional help should never be viewed as a sign of weakness, but as an act of self-preservation. Therapy provides a safe and confidential space to process trauma, develop healthy coping mechanisms, and address any underlying mental health concerns. It is a place where we can explore the deeper emotional impact of our experiences, offering a perspective beyond what a fellow paramedic or loved one might offer. It provides an opportunity for professional guidance, helping to identify, address, and manage potential mental health concerns effectively.

Engaging in activities outside of work that bring us joy and relaxation is crucial for maintaining a healthy work-life balance. This could range from spending time in nature, pursuing hobbies, engaging in social activities, or dedicating time to family and friends. These activities are not mere distractions; they are vital components in our overall well-being, serving as counterpoints to the often intense and emotionally draining aspects of our professional lives. Prioritizing these activities shows commitment to a balanced life, critical for sustaining our mental and physical fortitude.

Self-care for paramedics is not a one-size-fits-all proposition. It's a continuous journey of self-discovery, requiring experimentation and adaptation to find what works best for each individual. It involves a commitment to prioritizing our well-being, recognizing that our capacity to help others depends on our ability to care for ourselves first. It's about creating a sustainable lifestyle, weaving together physical fitness, mindfulness practices, healthy eating habits, adequate sleep, and strong social support. This holistic approach is not a luxury but an essential strategy for ensuring a long and fulfilling career in a demanding and challenging profession. It's about building a resilience that extends beyond the calls, allowing us to live full, meaningful lives, both on and off the ambulance.

The previous sections highlighted the importance of proactive self-care strategies in navigating the demanding world of paramedicine. However, even the most dedicated self-care routine can't entirely mitigate the cumulative stress, trauma, and emotional toll inherent in this profession. This is where seeking external support becomes crucial – a vital complement to, not a replacement for, personal strategies. Recognizing the need for help isn't a sign of weakness; it's a testament to self-awareness and a commitment to long-term well-being.

One of the most powerful resources available to paramedics is the peer support network. Sharing experiences with colleagues who understand the unique challenges of the job provides a sense of validation and camaraderie that's often invaluable. The shared understanding, the unspoken language of a difficult call, the silent nod of recognition – these are powerful tools in the fight against isolation. I recall a particularly brutal shift involving a pediatric trauma; the subsequent debrief with my partner wasn't a clinical discussion, but a shared space of vulnerability, allowing us to process the emotional aftermath. That shared experience, that unspoken understanding, created a bond stronger than any training exercise could forge.

Many emergency services organizations now offer formal peer support programs, providing structured environments for processing traumatic events and offering a confidential space for emotional support. These programs frequently employ trained peer support specialists – often fellow paramedics – who understand the nuances of the profession and can offer empathetic guidance and practical coping strategies. They aren't therapists, but they provide a crucial bridge, a connection to formal support systems. They can often identify warning signs of burnout, depression, or PTSD, encouraging timely intervention. The anonymity these programs offer often allows individuals to open up about their struggles without fear of professional repercussions.

Beyond peer support, most emergency medical services (EMS) organizations offer Employee Assistance Programs (EAPs). These programs provide confidential counseling, referral services, and other resources to help employees manage stress, work-life balance, and mental health concerns. EAPs are often overlooked, a hidden gem within the larger support structure. Their accessibility and confidentiality make them an invaluable asset. They offer a range of services, from short-term counseling sessions to referrals to specialists in areas like PTSD or substance abuse. The services are often free or offered at a significantly reduced cost, removing the significant financial barrier that can prevent many from seeking help. It's essential to familiarize yourself with your organization's EAP and utilize its resources.

While peer support and EAPs provide valuable initial support, seeking professional help from a qualified mental health professional is frequently necessary. A therapist specializing in trauma-informed care can provide personalized strategies for managing the unique emotional challenges faced by paramedics. They can help process the complex emotions that arise from exposure to trauma, death, and suffering, fostering resilience and healthier coping mechanisms. They can help unpack the ethical dilemmas we frequently encounter, offering a framework for managing the moral injury that can be so insidious. It's crucial to remember that seeking professional help isn't a sign of weakness; it's an act of self-preservation and a commitment to maintaining professional competence.

The stigma associated with mental health issues within the paramedic profession remains a significant hurdle. The culture of stoicism, the "tough guy" mentality, can make it difficult for individuals to openly acknowledge and address their emotional struggles. This is slowly changing, though, as more organizations actively promote mental health awareness and provide accessible support services. Open conversations, a willingness to challenge traditional norms, and a culture that values well-being are critical steps in dismantling this harmful stigma. We need to create an environment where seeking help is normalized and encouraged, rather than viewed as a potential career detriment.

The resources listed above are not exhaustive; various other avenues of support exist. Support groups specifically designed for paramedics provide a unique sense of community, allowing individuals to connect with others who understand the specific challenges of the job. These groups can offer a safe space to share experiences, share coping strategies, and foster a sense of belonging. Online forums and communities offer another avenue for connection and support, bridging geographical distances and providing a sense of collective experience. Many organizations also offer training workshops specifically designed for stress management, resilience building, and trauma processing. Actively seeking out and engaging with these resources is a crucial part of maintaining a healthy, fulfilling career.

Beyond formal support systems, building a strong support network outside of work is equally crucial. This might involve family, friends, or mentors who provide emotional support and understanding. They can offer a non-work-related perspective, a much-needed counterbalance to the emotionally demanding nature of the job. A non-judgmental ear, a shoulder to lean on, a trusted confidant – these relationships are essential components of maintaining a holistic approach to well-being. It is also vital to nurture these non-professional relationships, scheduling time specifically for relaxation and connection.

Finally, self-advocacy plays a crucial role in accessing and utilizing available resources. This involves actively identifying your own needs, communicating them effectively, and seeking out the support that best meets those needs. It's a proactive approach, taking control of your well-being. It might mean setting boundaries at work to protect your mental health, proactively seeking peer support following a particularly challenging call, or scheduling a therapy appointment before stress escalates.

Self-care is a journey, not a destination. It's a continuous process of self-discovery, adapting strategies as needed. It involves acknowledging that seeking support isn't a weakness; it's a sign of strength, a commitment to long-term health and well-being. The resources are available; the crucial step is actively seeking them out and making use of them. The ability to offer effective and compassionate care to our patients depends on our ability to care for ourselves first. By utilizing available support systems and openly engaging in self-advocacy, we can build a more resilient and supportive paramedic profession, allowing us to serve our communities effectively and maintain fulfilling lives both on and off the ambulance. This is not simply about extending our careers; it's about protecting our mental health, strengthening our relationships and fostering a sense of overall well-being – essential for a life lived fully and meaningfully. The paramedic profession demands much of us; in return, let us prioritize our own well-being, embracing the resources designed to support and sustain us.

The relentless pace of paramedicine, the constant exposure to suffering, death, and the ethical complexities of life-or-death decisions, creates a unique and potent cocktail of stressors. It's a job that demands resilience, a capacity to bounce back from adversity, to adapt to the unpredictable, and to maintain a sense of purpose and well-being amidst the chaos. Building this resilience isn't about becoming impervious to stress; it's about developing healthy coping mechanisms that allow you to navigate the inevitable challenges while preserving your mental and emotional health.

One of the most effective strategies I've found is mindfulness. It's more than just meditation, although that can be a powerful component. Mindfulness is about cultivating a present-moment awareness, focusing on the here and now rather than dwelling on the past or anxiously anticipating the future. On a chaotic scene, this might mean focusing on your breathing, grounding yourself in the present moment, and performing your tasks with deliberate intention. Between calls, it involves cultivating a sense of presence in your daily life— savoring a meal, fully engaging in a conversation, appreciating the simple pleasures that life offers. Mindfulness helps to break the cycle of rumination, that relentless replaying of stressful events, that can be so detrimental to mental health.

I remember one particularly challenging night. We had a series of traumatic calls – a multi-vehicle accident, a pediatric cardiac arrest, a violent assault – all within a few hours. By the end of the shift, I felt completely drained, emotionally raw. Instead of going straight home, I sat in my car for a few minutes, practicing deep, slow breaths. I focused on the feel of the steering wheel, the sounds around me, the sensation of the air on my skin. It was a small act, a few minutes stolen from the chaos, but it made a profound difference. It helped to create a sense of calm amidst the storm. It allowed me to transition from the intensity of the calls to the quiet solitude of my drive home.

Beyond mindfulness, physical self-care is undeniably crucial. This isn't about achieving some unattainable ideal of physical perfection; it's about engaging in regular activities that nourish your body and mind. Regular exercise, even a brisk walk or a short workout, can significantly reduce stress levels and improve mood. It's a natural mood booster, releasing endorphins that counteract the negative effects of chronic stress. Adequate sleep is equally important, something many paramedics struggle to achieve with unpredictable schedules and irregular shift patterns. Aim for a consistent sleep schedule, a routine that establishes a rhythm that can provide a safe haven from the chaotic shifts. Prioritizing healthy eating habits, avoiding excessive caffeine and alcohol, and staying hydrated, all work together to support overall well-being. They're small steps, but they form a significant foundation of self-care.

However, self-care strategies are only one piece of the puzzle. A balanced approach to resilience building necessitates a combination of individual strategies, external support, and a systemic approach to well-being within the EMS environment requires that we acknowledge that being a paramedic, in all its glory and trauma, significantly shapes one's identity. The job is intensely social, inherently interwoven with the lives of others, both colleagues and the patients we serve. We must acknowledge that this shapes who we are, how we experience the world, and what we prioritize in our lives.

Developing healthy coping mechanisms is crucial. This could involve anything from journaling to engaging in hobbies, spending time in nature, or connecting with loved ones. Journaling can be especially helpful in processing emotions, identifying triggers, and tracking progress in managing stress. For me, spending time in the woods, hiking or simply sitting by a stream, provides a sense of peace and perspective that is essential to decompressing after a stressful shift.

One of the most overlooked aspects of resilience building is setting healthy boundaries. This involves protecting your time, energy, and emotional resources. It's about saying "no" to additional shifts when you're feeling overwhelmed, taking breaks during long shifts, or setting limits on work-related discussions outside of work hours. Establishing boundaries is an act of self-preservation; it's about valuing your own mental and physical health. This often means learning to say "no", to accept that you cannot always be available and always capable of offering a perfect solution. This is particularly important after challenging experiences – the need to disconnect, to recharge your energies, becomes paramount.

The importance of a strong support system cannot be overstated. This includes friends, family, and colleagues who understand the challenges of the job and can offer emotional support, empathy, and a listening ear. It's important to cultivate and nurture these relationships; they're a lifeline during difficult times. It's equally crucial to actively engage with other paramedics, to allow ourselves to be vulnerable and open about our experiences. Creating an environment within our teams that supports this sharing is critical.

The professional support available needs to be explored and engaged. This isn't a sign of weakness; it's an act of self-preservation. Utilizing employee assistance programs (EAPs), peer support networks, and mental health professionals are all crucial elements of resilience building. These resources provide a safe and confidential space to process traumatic experiences, receive guidance, and develop coping strategies. I've found that sharing my experiences with a therapist specializing in trauma-informed care has been instrumental in helping me process the cumulative effects of years on the job.

However, accessing and utilizing these resources isn't always easy. The stigma surrounding mental health in emergency services is a persistent and significant challenge. A culture of stoicism, a reluctance to admit vulnerability, can create significant barriers. This culture needs to change; open conversations about mental health need to be normalized. We, as a profession, need to foster an environment where seeking help is viewed as an act of strength, not weakness. This requires leadership within EMS organizations to actively promote mental health awareness, providing training and resources to support paramedics. It means normalizing conversations about our vulnerabilities.

Moreover, there's a critical need for increased training and education on resilience building strategies within paramedic training programs. Integrating mindfulness techniques, stress management skills, and trauma-informed care into the curriculum can equip new paramedics with the tools they need to thrive in this challenging profession from the outset. It's about preventative care, building a foundation of resilience early on to mitigate the impact of cumulative stress and trauma.

Furthermore, organizations must actively promote a culture of well-being. This involves prioritizing mental health initiatives, providing access to mental health services, and creating a supportive and inclusive work environment. Creating a culture where open dialogue is supported, where asking for help doesn't carry risk, is absolutely essential. It's a systemic issue that requires a systemic solution. It involves leaders championing mental well-being, creating resources that reduce the barriers, and creating environments that truly support their staff.

Ultimately, building resilience is a continuous process, a journey, not a destination. It's about ongoing self-reflection, self-care, and seeking support when needed. It's about recognizing our own limitations, allowing ourselves to be vulnerable and creating spaces and networks where we can collectively support one another and build resilience within our ranks. It's about accepting the emotional toll of this job and having the resources to manage it effectively, to navigate the challenging aspects while prioritizing our own well-being, not just for our own sake, but for the sake of the quality of our lives and our ability to serve our communities. By investing in our own resilience, we invest in the future of paramedicine, creating a more sustainable and supportive profession where everyone can thrive, both on and off the ambulance.

4

After the Shift: Processing Trauma

The emotional residue of a traumatic call can linger long after the sirens have faded and the adrenaline has subsided. It's not simply a matter of "shaking it off" – the images, the sounds, the sheer weight of human suffering can become deeply embedded in our minds and bodies. This is where the crucial work of processing trauma begins. It's a deeply personal journey, and the path to healing will look different for everyone. But certain strategies consistently prove their worth in helping paramedics navigate this complex terrain.

One of the most effective, yet often overlooked, tools is journaling. It's a simple act – putting pen to paper, or fingers to keyboard – but its therapeutic power is significant. Journaling isn't about crafting perfect prose; it's about releasing the emotions that are bottled up inside. It's a safe space to articulate the raw, unfiltered experiences of the day, to confront the difficult emotions without judgment. I've found that simply writing down the details of a particularly challenging call – the patient's story, my own reactions, the thoughts that raced through my mind – can help to externalize the trauma, to lessen its grip on my psyche. The act of describing the events, however painful, can begin to unravel their power over me. It provides a structured way to process these experiences; it allows me to separate myself slightly from the immediate emotional intensity. It allows for reflection, not rumination.

Sometimes, what emerges from the pages is surprisingly insightful. Patterns begin to emerge, underlying anxieties and recurring themes reveal themselves. These insights can then be used to develop targeted coping strategies. For example, I discovered through journaling that certain types of calls – pediatric emergencies, in particular – were disproportionately affecting me. Recognizing this pattern allowed me to proactively address my responses to these situations, developing specific mindfulness techniques to manage my emotional reactions.

But journaling alone isn't always enough. For many paramedics, seeking professional help is a crucial step in the healing process. Therapy, particularly trauma-informed therapy, provides a safe and supportive space to process complex emotions, explore underlying coping mechanisms, and develop healthier strategies for managing stress. A good therapist understands the unique challenges faced by first responders, offering a non-judgmental ear and providing guidance tailored to the profession's specific demands. This isn't a sign of weakness; it's an act of self-preservation. It's an acknowledgement that we are human, susceptible to the emotional toll of the job, and that seeking help isn't just acceptable but essential.

I remember a colleague who initially resisted seeking therapy. He felt a strong sense of shame and inadequacy, believing that a strong paramedic should be able to handle anything. But after months of struggling in silence, battling recurring nightmares and experiencing significant anxiety, he finally reached out for help. The transformation was remarkable. He learned to identify his triggers, to develop healthier coping strategies, and to build a stronger sense of self-compassion. His experience highlights the importance of breaking down the stigma surrounding mental health within our profession. It takes courage to ask for help, but the rewards are immense.

Mindfulness practices, as previously discussed, remain incredibly valuable tools in navigating the aftermath of traumatic events. These practices, including meditation, deep breathing exercises, and mindful movement, help to regulate the nervous system, reducing the intensity of emotional responses and promoting a sense of calm. It's not about escaping the difficult emotions; it's about learning to approach them with greater awareness and compassion. The practice of mindfulness allows me to observe my thoughts and feelings without judgment, to recognize them as transient experiences rather than permanent fixtures of my identity. This detachment, this ability to observe rather than be consumed by emotion, is critical in processing trauma.

The specific techniques of mindfulness can be tailored to individual needs. Some paramedics find guided meditations helpful, while others prefer simpler practices like focusing on their breath during stressful moments or engaging in mindful walks in nature. The key is to find what works best for you and to integrate these practices into your daily routine. Consistency is key – even short periods of mindfulness can make a significant difference over time. The cumulative effect is a profound sense of inner peace, a resilience that can weather the storms of the job.

Beyond professional support and individual practices, building a strong support system is critical. This isn't just about having friends and family; it's about cultivating genuine connections with colleagues who understand the unique challenges of paramedic work. Sharing experiences with fellow paramedics, knowing that you're not alone in the emotional toll, can be incredibly powerful. Peer support networks, often found within EMS agencies or professional organizations, provide a safe and confidential space for paramedics to connect, share their experiences, and offer each other emotional support.

Many organizations offer Employee Assistance Programs (EAPs), providing access to confidential counseling and other resources. These programs offer a valuable resource, offering a bridge to mental health support and sometimes providing referrals to specialized professionals experienced in working with first responders. These EAPs frequently offer a range of services, including individual and group therapy, stress management workshops, and access to various community resources. They offer a critical safety net, helping paramedics navigate challenging emotional periods without incurring the added stress of financial burdens.

However, accessing these resources shouldn't be viewed as a solitary act. Colleagues, supervisors, and agency leadership play a critical role in promoting a culture of support and destigmatizing mental health issues within the profession. This requires a collective shift in mindset, moving away from outdated notions of stoicism and toward a more open and compassionate approach. It's a matter of recognizing that mental health is just as important as physical health. The health of our teams hinges on a commitment to supporting each other, both emotionally and professionally.

The long-term effects of cumulative trauma can be significant, leading to burnout, compassion fatigue, and even post-traumatic stress disorder (PTSD). It's essential to recognize that these aren't merely temporary setbacks; they are potential consequences of the job that demand active attention and intervention. Recognizing the symptoms early is vital; early intervention can greatly improve outcomes and reduce the impact of chronic stress.

Regular self-assessment is key. This involves paying attention to changes in mood, sleep patterns, appetite, and energy levels. If you notice significant shifts in any of these areas, it's crucial to seek professional help. Don't wait until you're at breaking point; proactive care is much more effective than crisis intervention.

Beyond individual strategies, systemic changes are needed within the EMS community to support the mental health of paramedics. This includes investing in comprehensive training programs that equip paramedics with effective coping mechanisms from the outset of their careers. It also requires creating a workplace culture that normalizes seeking help, fostering open communication about mental health, and providing readily accessible resources. This involves organizational leadership making a commitment to support the well-being of their staff, actively promoting mental health initiatives, and ensuring that adequate resources are available.

Ultimately, processing trauma is a continuous process, requiring ongoing self-reflection, proactive self-care, and a willingness to seek support when needed. It's a journey, not a destination, demanding a multifaceted approach that combines individual resilience-building strategies, accessible professional resources, and a supportive organizational culture. By prioritizing our mental and emotional well-being, we are not only safeguarding our own health but also ensuring the sustainability and effectiveness of the entire paramedic profession. We're not just treating patients; we're investing in a future where our teams can thrive in both the demanding field and the quiet moments of reflection that follow.

Moral injury is a wound to the soul, a silent suffering that often goes unrecognized in the high-pressure world of emergency medical services. Unlike post-traumatic stress disorder (PTSD), which stems from witnessing or experiencing trauma, moral injury arises from perpetrating, witnessing, or failing to prevent acts that violate one's deeply held moral beliefs. For paramedics, this can manifest in countless ways, leaving a profound and lasting impact on our well-being.

One of the most common sources of moral injury for paramedics is the experience of witnessing preventable deaths. I recall a call involving a young child who had been in a car accident. Despite our best efforts, we were unable to save the child's life. The scene was chaotic, filled with the screams of family members and the emotional toll on the first responders at the scene was significant. The child's life could have been saved if the parents had been more diligent in child safety practices. The haunting image of the child's lifeless body, coupled with the knowledge that the tragedy might have been preventable, ignited a deep sense of moral failure that has stayed with me. This feeling of helplessness, of having been unable to prevent a tragedy, eats away at your conscience. It's a profound feeling of failure, even if objectively nothing more could have been done. It's the "what ifs" and "could have beens" that relentlessly replay in the mind, undermining our confidence and fueling feelings of guilt and inadequacy.

Another prevalent source of moral injury is the perception of inadequate resources or systemic failures that compromise patient care. We've all been there, facing situations where a lack of equipment, understaffing, or bureaucratic red tape impeded our ability to provide optimal care. The frustration and anger that boils over in these moments can lead to a sense of moral compromise – a feeling that we failed to live up to our professional oath because the system failed us. I once responded to a call in a rural area where the nearest hospital was over an hour away. The patient required immediate intervention but due to logistical constraints and distance we couldn't adequately aid the patient in time. The delay directly impacted the patient's outcome, and the sense of helplessness born from this systemic failure continues to haunt me. This isn't about individual blame; it's about the inherent moral conflict that arises when our commitment to providing the best possible care is hampered by external factors beyond our control.

These situations can lead to profound emotional distress, impacting our personal lives and professional effectiveness. The symptoms of moral injury can be subtle or overwhelming, manifesting as persistent feelings of guilt, shame, anger, betrayal, or even numbness. These feelings can spill over into other aspects of our lives, affecting our relationships, sleep, appetite, and overall mental health. We might find ourselves constantly replaying the events in our heads, searching for answers that may not exist, constantly dissecting the choices we made, second-guessing our every action. The critical self-analysis may become self-destructive rumination.

Addressing moral injury requires a multi-pronged approach. While journaling and mindfulness techniques remain important, they alone may not suffice to address the deep-seated moral conflicts at play. It requires confronting the root of the issue and actively seeking help to process the underlying emotions. This often involves seeking professional help from therapists experienced in treating moral injury in first responders. These therapists are trained to create a safe space for open discussion, to help us acknowledge our feelings, and to guide us towards constructive coping strategies. They can help us understand that these feelings are normal and valid responses to extraordinary circumstances, and to help us process the emotional load. They can help to prevent a spiral into depression or PTSD. Open conversations with colleagues who understand the unique stressors faced by paramedics can be invaluable in this process. It helps to know that we aren't alone in our struggles and that others share similar experiences. Sharing experiences without judgment is critical to healing.

Additionally, working towards systemic change within the EMS community is crucial. This involves advocating for improved resource allocation, better staffing levels, and more efficient systems to reduce preventable delays in care. This isn't just about providing better working conditions; it's about upholding the fundamental ethical values of the profession. This includes promoting a culture of open communication, encouraging peer support, and reducing the stigma around seeking professional help for mental health concerns.

There's a pervasive culture within emergency services of stoicism and suppressing emotion. We are expected to be strong, resilient, and always capable of handling any situation. However, ignoring our emotional needs and refusing to acknowledge the moral dilemmas we face will only exacerbate the problem. We need to move toward a culture that embraces vulnerability and prioritizes the mental health and emotional well-being of its members. This requires a concerted effort from all levels – individual paramedics, supervisors, and agency leadership. Training programs should specifically address moral injury, equipping paramedics with the tools and resources needed to navigate these complex ethical issues from the start of their careers. It needs to be normalized and embedded into the culture. Regular debriefing sessions, led by trained professionals, can also provide a safe space to process challenging calls and address underlying moral concerns.

But what about the individual? What steps can each of us take to begin healing from the wounds of moral injury? It starts with self-awareness – acknowledging the emotional impact of the profession and recognizing the signs of moral injury in ourselves and in our colleagues. It involves taking proactive steps to build resilience, developing healthy coping mechanisms that are sustainable and not just a short-term fix.

Remember that guilt and shame are common responses, but they are not your identity. Moral injury can lead to a sense of being morally tainted, but these feelings are not inherently true. We are not defined by our mistakes, but by our commitment to learning and growing from them. This requires self-compassion. Treating ourselves with the same kindness and understanding we would offer a struggling colleague is vital in navigating this difficult emotional landscape.

This also entails actively engaging in self-care practices that nurture our physical and mental health. Physical exercise, healthy diet, sufficient sleep – these may seem like simple aspects, but they're foundational building blocks of a strong, resilient self. These are not simply nice-to-haves but essential for managing the inherent stresses and emotional tolls of the profession. We cannot pour from an empty cup.

Developing a strong support network outside of work is also crucial. This could involve family, friends, or support groups specifically designed for first responders. These connections provide a safe space to process emotions and to feel understood, and offer non-judgmental validation that is critical for healing.

Ultimately, healing from moral injury is a journey, not a destination. It is a long and arduous process, requiring patience, self-compassion, and a willingness to seek professional help. The road to recovery may be long and winding, with setbacks along the way, but with support and continued self-reflection, we can find a path towards healing and regain a sense of wholeness. The dedication of emergency services must extend to the well-being of its professionals. Addressing moral injury is not merely a matter of improving individual well-being; it's about safeguarding the ethical foundations of our profession and ensuring that those who dedicate their lives to saving others have the support they need to heal from the invisible wounds they carry. Only then can we truly serve our communities with compassion, integrity, and unwavering commitment.

Burnout in emergency medical services (EMS) isn't merely a matter of exhaustion; it's a systemic erosion of one's physical, emotional, and mental well-being, a slow simmering that can ultimately extinguish the flame of passion and dedication that initially drew us to this profession. It's a creeping malaise, often insidious in its onset, manifesting as apathy, cynicism, and a profound sense of detachment from the work that once fueled us. It's a dangerous and often overlooked consequence of a job that demands constant vigilance, unwavering commitment, and an almost superhuman capacity for empathy.

I remember a colleague, a veteran paramedic with over two decades of experience, who suddenly started making careless mistakes. He, once a paragon of precision and calm under pressure, began exhibiting lapses in judgment, his sharp wit replaced by a weary silence. His normally vibrant energy had been replaced by a palpable exhaustion that permeated every interaction. He'd become detached, almost robotic in his responses to calls. It wasn't a sudden crisis; it was a gradual decline, a slow unraveling that went largely unnoticed until it became impossible to ignore. His burnout wasn't a sudden event; it was a cumulative effect of years of relentless pressure, relentless emotional demands, and a profound lack of self-care.

Preventing burnout isn't about achieving some mythical state of perpetual energy; it's about cultivating a sustainable approach to the profession, one that acknowledges the inherent emotional and physical demands while prioritizing personal well-being. It's about building a life – not just a career – that can withstand the intense pressures of this profession. This requires a proactive and multi-faceted strategy, encompassing elements of workload management, boundary setting, and a conscious commitment to self-care.

Workload management is often the first line of defense against burnout. This isn't simply about reducing the number of hours worked; it's about a more nuanced approach to how we engage with our work. Learning to say "no" to extra shifts or calls when feeling overwhelmed is paramount. It's accepting that we have limitations, that we are not superhuman, and that prioritizing our own well-being is not a sign of weakness, but of self-preservation. This may necessitate difficult conversations with supervisors, but asserting our boundaries is essential for preserving our long-term health and well-being.

Effective time management is equally critical. This entails prioritizing tasks, delegating when possible, and learning to let go of perfectionism – a particularly challenging aspect for many of us in the EMS profession. Perfectionism, while seemingly a positive trait, can be a significant contributor to burnout. The constant striving for flawlessness can lead to overwhelming stress, anxiety, and an inability to disconnect from work even outside of shifts. Embracing imperfection is a necessary and liberating step towards a more sustainable career. It's acknowledging that we are human, that we will inevitably make mistakes, and that these mistakes are opportunities for growth, not reasons for self-recrimination.

Beyond workload management, setting healthy boundaries between professional and personal life is crucial. This involves establishing clear separation between work and home life, actively disengaging from work-related stressors during personal time, and safeguarding personal time for activities that nurture our well-being. This might involve disconnecting from work emails and messages during off-hours, dedicating specific times to family and friends, or engaging in hobbies that offer respite from the constant demands of the job. For me, disconnecting after a particularly challenging shift often involves a long run. The physical exertion provides a cathartic release of tension, clearing my mind and allowing me to process the events of the shift without feeling constantly overwhelmed.

Prioritizing self-care shouldn't be seen as a luxury; it's a necessity, a non-negotiable component of long-term well-being in this profession. Self-care is not just about pampering; it's a multifaceted approach that encompasses physical, mental, and emotional health. It's about taking concrete steps to improve our overall well-being. This includes maintaining a healthy diet, engaging in regular physical exercise, prioritizing sufficient sleep, and practicing mindfulness techniques. These may seem like simple actions, but they are fundamental building blocks of resilience. They are the preventative maintenance that keeps our emotional and physical engines running smoothly.

Mindfulness, in particular, has been profoundly beneficial in my own life. Learning to be present in the moment, to focus on my breath, and to let go of anxieties about the future or regrets about the past has dramatically reduced my overall stress levels. It's a constant practice, one that requires dedication and patience, but the rewards are significant. It allows me to process difficult calls more effectively, to detach from the emotional weight of my work, and to experience a greater sense of calm and equanimity in my life.

Building a strong support network is also essential. This involves cultivating meaningful relationships with colleagues, family, and friends who understand the unique challenges of working in EMS. These connections provide a sense of community, validation, and support, counteracting the feelings of isolation that often accompany the profession. It's essential to share our experiences, both the triumphs and the tragedies, with those who can offer empathy and understanding without judgment. Finding a mentor or a peer who shares the same career trajectory can be incredibly valuable.

However, it's crucial to recognize that seeking professional support is not a sign of weakness, but a sign of strength. Therapists specializing in first responders are uniquely positioned to help us navigate the emotional complexities of our profession. They provide a safe space to process difficult experiences, to develop healthy coping mechanisms, and to build resilience in the face of adversity. It is vital that we, as a profession, remove the stigma surrounding seeking professional help. It is a sign of strength and self-awareness, not a weakness.

Regular debriefing sessions, both formal and informal, also play a crucial role in burnout prevention. These sessions, whether led by a trained professional or among colleagues, provide an opportunity to process challenging calls, to share experiences, and to normalize the difficult emotions that accompany our work. It's in these shared moments of vulnerability that we discover we're not alone in our struggles, that we can find strength in shared experience, and that we can collectively cultivate a culture of support and understanding.

Ultimately, preventing burnout is an ongoing process, a commitment to nurturing our well-being on multiple levels. It demands an awareness of our limits, a willingness to set boundaries, and a proactive approach to self-care. By prioritizing these strategies, we are not merely safeguarding our individual well-being; we are strengthening the very fabric of our profession, ensuring that we can continue to provide the compassionate and effective care that our communities deserve for years to come.

The dedication and commitment we show to our patients must extend to ourselves. We must be our own advocates, prioritizing our mental and emotional health alongside our professional skills. The future of emergency services rests not only on our technical proficiency but on our capacity for self-preservation.

The relentless pace, the emotional toll, the constant exposure to trauma – these are all realities of paramedic work that can lead to burnout, and sometimes, the need for a significant career shift. But the skills honed in the field aren't confined to the back of an ambulance. In fact, the adaptability, resilience, and critical thinking abilities developed as a paramedic translate surprisingly well to a wide array of alternative career paths. Recognizing this opens up a world of possibilities for those seeking a change, allowing them to leverage their experience and expertise in new and rewarding ways.

One of the most obvious transitions involves moving into roles within the healthcare system. The experience gained managing critical situations, providing immediate medical intervention, and dealing with high-pressure environments is highly valuable in various hospital settings. Consider the potential for a transition into emergency room nursing. The knowledge of rapid assessment, emergency procedures, and medication administration directly aligns with the responsibilities of an ER nurse. The ability to stay calm and make life-saving decisions under intense pressure is equally critical in both professions.

Furthermore, paramedics often find themselves well-suited for roles in urgent care clinics or occupational health. Urgent care often requires the quick assessment and triage of patients, skills paramedics already possess. In occupational health, the ability to assess injuries, provide first aid, and develop preventative strategies is highly beneficial. The ability to conduct thorough patient assessments, determine the urgency of their conditions, and communicate effectively with medical personnel is fundamental to both paramedic and urgent care roles. One of my colleagues transitioned into occupational health after years in the field, finding the shift to a less demanding but still impactful role rewarding.

The transferable skills aren't limited to direct patient care, either. The leadership, communication, and teamwork honed on the job are highly sought after in various management and training positions. Paramedics frequently lead teams, make critical decisions under immense pressure, and communicate effectively with patients, families, and other medical professionals. These skills are highly valued in supervisory roles within EMS itself, but also translate into roles in other sectors, such as project management, operations management, or even teaching.

For instance, the ability to mentor and train new paramedics is a natural transition for seasoned professionals. Sharing knowledge, passing on practical skills, and fostering a sense of teamwork become essential components of a training role. The experience of handling diverse situations, adapting to changing circumstances, and communicating effectively in stressful situations makes paramedics ideal candidates for training programs across the board. I've seen several colleagues successfully transition into this path, finding fulfillment in shaping the next generation of paramedics. They found their existing expertise valuable in creating a supportive and rigorous training environment.

Moving outside of healthcare altogether is also a viable option. The problem-solving skills, the quick decision-making abilities, and the resilience developed as a paramedic are highly valuable in numerous fields. Consider, for instance, the potential for a transition into roles requiring high levels of responsibility and quick thinking. The ability to react effectively under stress is a key asset in security, law enforcement, or even firefighting. These roles involve similar elements of risk assessment, rapid response, and teamwork. The ability to remain calm in critical situations is not easily taught, and it's a skill paramedics inherently possess.

Moreover, the intense focus on details, the ability to remain calm under pressure, and the effective communication skills honed in the field can lead to successful careers in fields as diverse as risk management, safety training, or even technical writing. The capacity to analyze situations, identify potential hazards, and explain complex issues clearly is crucial in these sectors. The ability to translate complex information into understandable terms, which is a daily requirement for a paramedic interacting with patients, families, and other professionals, is highly transferable.

For paramedics considering a career transition, it's essential to carefully assess their strengths and interests. Identifying the skills they wish to utilize in a new career path is the first step. This often involves reflecting on the aspects of their paramedic career they enjoyed the most and the skills they utilized most effectively. Are they passionate about teaching and mentoring? Do they excel in leadership roles? Do they thrive in fast-paced, high-pressure environments? Answering these questions provides a roadmap for exploring potential career paths.

Networking plays a crucial role in the transition process. Connecting with individuals in different fields, attending industry events, and utilizing online platforms like LinkedIn can help to uncover hidden opportunities and provide insights into different career paths. Talking to people already working in alternative professions can offer valuable perspectives and guidance. Many professionals are happy to share their career journeys and offer advice to those considering a similar path. This personal connection can be invaluable in navigating the transition.

Finally, don't underestimate the value of further education or training. Depending on the desired career path, additional qualifications may be necessary to enhance competitiveness. However, the foundational skills and experience gained as a paramedic often serve as a strong basis for further learning. This can range from specialized medical certifications to courses in leadership, management, or other relevant fields.

The transition from paramedic to another profession isn't always easy, but it's often profoundly rewarding. It's an opportunity to leverage the unique skills and experience gained in a demanding and often challenging career while pursuing a new path aligned with personal goals and well-being. The experiences, both positive and negative, shape and strengthen the paramedic, providing a solid foundation for future success, no matter the chosen career. It's a testament to the resilience and adaptability that define those who dedicate themselves to this profession. The skills that make for a great paramedic are highly valuable, applicable, and highly sought after in a remarkably wide range of fields. The transition might involve challenges, but the potential for a fulfilling and successful career in a new direction is substantial and often surprisingly accessible. The support networks we build in the EMS profession are valuable, and keeping those connections can aid in the transition. The community is there to lend a hand and offer guidance. The journey after the shift can be a journey of growth and discovery, leading to new and fulfilling opportunities.

Leaving the adrenaline-fueled world of emergency response doesn't mean severing ties with the paramedic community. In fact, the skills and experiences gained over years of service translate beautifully into opportunities to contribute meaningfully, shaping the future of the profession and supporting those who follow in our footsteps. The transition from active duty to a role of mentorship, advocacy, or even research allows for a continued connection to the field, providing a sense of purpose and fulfillment beyond the immediate demands of emergency calls.

One of the most rewarding ways to contribute is through mentorship. The wisdom gained from years of experience, the countless calls witnessed, the lessons learned from both successes and failures – all of these form a rich tapestry of knowledge that can be invaluable to aspiring paramedics. Sharing this knowledge isn't just about imparting technical skills; it's about sharing the wisdom of the profession, the emotional resilience required to navigate the challenges, and the importance of ethical decision-making under pressure. I recall mentoring a young paramedic fresh out of training. She was incredibly skilled technically, but she lacked the confidence to handle the emotional weight of some calls. We spent hours discussing techniques for emotional processing, the importance of self-care, and recognizing her own limitations. Watching her grow in confidence and develop her own coping mechanisms was deeply satisfying. Mentoring provides a direct and tangible impact, nurturing the next generation of skilled and resilient para-medics. Mentorship can take various forms, from formal training programs to informal guidance and support. It can involve providing one-on-one coaching, leading workshops, or simply being a listening ear for someone navigating the complexities of the field.

Beyond formal mentorship, there are countless opportunities to contribute to the paramedic community through advocacy. Our unique perspective, gained from firsthand experience on the front lines, allows us to advocate for policies and practices that improve patient care and support paramedic well-being. This advocacy might involve working with local or national EMS associations, participating in legislative ini-tiatives, or simply raising awareness about the challenges faced by para-medics. For example, during a period of significant understaffing in our region, I worked with other paramedics to advocate for increased fund-ing and improved working conditions. We presented data highlighting the impact of burnout and high call volumes on patient safety and para-medic morale. This effort ultimately led to improved staffing levels and a renewed focus on paramedic well-being within the local EMS system. Advocacy might also involve speaking publicly about important issues, such as the need for improved mental health resources for paramedics, the importance of effective trauma response protocols, or the critical role of paramedics in disaster response.

Moreover, the rich dataset of experiences accumulated throughout a paramedic career presents unique opportunities for research. The field of prehospital emergency care is constantly evolving, and the insights gleaned from the daily realities of paramedic work can inform and im-prove practices. Paramedics have a unique vantage point on patient out-comes, challenges in prehospital care, and the effectiveness of various treatment strategies. This firsthand knowledge can be instrumental in shaping evidence-based practices and improving the overall quality of prehospital care. I've been involved in several research projects, focusing on the efficacy of different pain management techniques and the impact of various communication strategies on patient anxiety. Our findings have been published in peer-reviewed journals and have directly informed changes in our local EMS protocols. The opportunity to contribute to this type of research extends the scope of influence far beyond the immediate scope of a single individual's practice. The contribution of paramedics in research is vital for enhancing patient care, shaping policy, and improving the overall landscape of emergency medical services.

Contributing to the paramedic community isn't limited to these larger-scale endeavors. Smaller acts of support can be equally impactful. Simply offering encouragement and support to colleagues, sharing knowledge and resources, and maintaining a positive and collaborative work environment all contribute to a strong and resilient paramedic community. Sharing personal experiences, both positive and challenging, creates a sense of camaraderie and mutual understanding, mitigating feelings of isolation and helping individuals manage the unique stresses associated with the profession. This support network can be critical for both new paramedics and those nearing the end of their careers. I've seen firsthand the power of simple acts of kindness and mutual support in boosting morale and fostering resilience amongst my colleagues.

The emotional toll of paramedic work is often underestimated. The constant exposure to trauma, loss, and suffering can take a significant toll, leading to burnout and mental health challenges. Supporting each other in managing this emotional burden is a crucial aspect of maintaining a healthy and effective paramedic community. This includes creating a culture of open communication, where paramedics feel comfortable discussing their emotional struggles without fear of judgment. It also involves actively seeking and utilizing resources that promote mental health and well-being. This could involve establishing peer support programs, providing access to mental health professionals, or promoting self-care strategies. One of the most effective strategies I've witnessed is the creation of peer-support groups, where paramedics can share their experiences in a safe and non-judgmental environment. These groups provide a space for processing difficult emotions, sharing coping strategies, and building a strong sense of community.

Furthermore, contributing to the paramedic community can involve participation in community outreach programs and initiatives. This might involve providing CPR training, conducting injury prevention workshops, or participating in community health fairs. These activities not only educate the public about emergency medical care but also enhance the positive image of paramedics within the community and contribute to broader public health goals. These activities provide an opportunity to connect with the community, promote health education and awareness, and highlight the role of paramedics in improving public safety and health outcomes.

Another avenue for paramedics to leave a legacy is through the creation and sharing of educational materials. This can range from developing training materials for new paramedics to writing articles or books about paramedicine. These resources can serve to educate, inspire, and support future generations of paramedics. The process of creating such materials requires a deep reflection on one's experience and expertise, creating the perfect opportunity to both synthesize the learning acquired throughout one's career and ensure this knowledge is passed down to those who follow.

In conclusion, the journey of a paramedic doesn't end with the final shift. The skills, experiences, and empathy honed in the field offer valuable opportunities to contribute meaningfully to the paramedic community, shaping the future of the profession and supporting the well-being of those who serve. Whether through mentorship, advocacy, research, or simply supporting colleagues, the legacy of a paramedic can extend far beyond the emergency calls and extend to the lives and well-being of future generations of paramedics. The dedication and compassion we bring to the profession are not limited to the emergency room; these values can be extended to build and support a thriving paramedic community, strengthening the profession and improving the lives of countless individuals, long after the sirens have faded. The ongoing support and contributions of experienced paramedics are vital for the strength and evolution of prehospital emergency medical care. Leaving a legacy is not just about what we accomplish during our active years in the field, but also about the lasting positive impact we have on the community long after our shifts have ended.

5

The Tools of the Trade: Essential Equipment

The transition from the emotional and relational aspects of paramedicine to the technical domain might seem abrupt, but the two are inextricably linked. The effectiveness of our interventions hinges not just on our emotional intelligence and empathy, but also on our mastery of the sophisticated technology at our disposal. Advanced life support (ALS) equipment represents the cutting edge of prehospital care, a constant evolution of tools designed to improve patient outcomes in the most critical moments. Proficiency with these tools is paramount, requiring not only technical skill but also a deep understanding of their limitations and the potential for malfunction.

One of the cornerstones of modern ALS is the cardiac monitor/defibrillator. This seemingly simple box is a complex piece of technology capable of analyzing a patient's heart rhythm, delivering life-saving defibrillation shocks, and providing continuous ECG monitoring. The ability to interpret these rhythms quickly and accurately is critical. I remember a call involving a young athlete who collapsed on a soccer field. His rhythm initially appeared to be ventricular fibrillation (VF), a life-threatening arrhythmia. We immediately initiated CPR and delivered a defibrillatory shock. However, a closer examination of the rhythm revealed a rare form of polymorphic VT, which required a different treatment strategy. That call underscored the importance of continuous monitoring and the need for paramedics to have a strong foundational understanding of cardiac physiology. Misinterpreting a rhythm can have fatal consequences, highlighting the necessity of continuous professional development and ongoing training in advanced cardiac life support (ACLS).

Beyond rhythm interpretation, the cardiac monitor/defibrillator's capabilities extend to the measurement of other vital signs, such as heart rate, oxygen saturation (SpO2), and blood pressure. This integrated approach streamlines data collection, allowing paramedics to assess the patient's overall condition efficiently. Moreover, some devices offer sophisticated analysis features, providing waveform interpretation and diagnostic support. The data collected provides crucial information which informs our treatment decisions. This is especially important in situations where the patient might not be able to communicate their symptoms effectively. For instance, an elderly patient who has fallen and sustained a head injury may not be able to verbally describe their pain level or the extent of their injury. The objective data from the monitor, in conjunction with our clinical assessment, helps paint a complete picture and guide our treatment choices. Regular calibration and maintenance of these devices are non-negotiable, ensuring accuracy and reliability in these life-or-death situations.

Another crucial piece of ALS equipment is the automated external defibrillator (AED). While AEDs are often found in public places, their use on ambulances requires a more nuanced understanding of their capabilities and limitations. AEDs are designed for ease of use, primarily for non-medical personnel, but paramedics need to know how to interpret the device's prompts, address any technical malfunctions, and integrate AED use into a broader resuscitation strategy. The AED is not a standalone solution; it's a critical component of the entire resuscitation plan, which must include effective CPR, airway management, and advanced life support interventions. I've seen instances where AEDs have malfunctioned, requiring paramedics to troubleshoot the problem swiftly, or where a seemingly clear VF rhythm was actually a different rhythm requiring a different approach. The critical thinking and problem-solving skills required for these situations cannot be overstated.

Intubation and airway management represent another critical facet of ALS. Paramedics often use advanced airway devices, such as endotracheal tubes (ETTs), laryngeal masks (LMA), and other supraglottic airway devices, to ensure a patent airway. These tools demand a high level of technical expertise and proficiency. Successful intubation relies not only on technical skill but also on a thorough understanding of anatomy, physiology, and potential complications. Improper intubation can lead to serious complications, such as esophageal intubation or airway trauma. Regular training and practice are vital to maintain proficiency. The use of video laryngoscopes has transformed airway management in recent years, allowing for a clearer view of the airway and improving the success rate of intubation, particularly in challenging situations. Furthermore, the integration of capnography, which measures carbon dioxide levels in exhaled breath, provides real-time feedback on the proper placement of the endotracheal tube.

Fluid resuscitation is another critical ALS intervention, often involving the administration of intravenous (IV) fluids or intraosseous (IO) access. IV access is a common procedure for paramedics, but obtaining effective IV access can be challenging, particularly in patients who are dehydrated, hypovolemic, or have fragile veins. IO access provides an alternative route for fluid administration, especially valuable in pediatric patients or those with limited venous access. However, IO access requires specialized training and a sound understanding of appropriate insertion sites and potential complications. The choice between IV and IO access is determined by a number of factors, including patient age, clinical status, and the urgency of fluid resuscitation. Moreover, the selection of the appropriate fluid solution depends on the patient's underlying condition. Overly aggressive fluid resuscitation can itself lead to complications, demonstrating the importance of careful monitoring and titration.

Advanced life support also includes the administration of medications. Paramedics carry a range of medications, ranging from analgesics and antiemetics to advanced medications, such as vasopressors and sedatives. The appropriate selection and administration of medication requires a thorough understanding of pharmacology and a consideration of potential drug interactions and adverse effects. Moreover, accurate dosage calculation and safe administration techniques are crucial. This underscores the need for continuous professional development in pharmacology and a commitment to staying current with best practices.

Beyond individual pieces of equipment, the integration of technology into the modern ambulance itself plays a critical role. The integration of electronic patient care records (ePCRs) has streamlined documentation and improved data collection. These systems often include built-in diagnostic support tools and decision-making aids, offering paramedics guidance in complex clinical situations. Mobile data terminals (MDTs) allow for real-time communication with hospitals and dispatch centers, facilitating seamless handoff of patient care and optimizing resource allocation. Navigation systems built into ambulances improve response times, while integrated telemedicine capabilities allow for remote consultations with specialists, providing additional expertise in challenging cases.

Finally, maintaining the equipment itself is a crucial part of ensuring its effective use. Regular preventative maintenance and prompt repair are vital for the safe and reliable functioning of all ALS equipment. This includes regular calibration checks, battery replacements, and software updates. The failure of a piece of equipment at a critical moment can have severe consequences, emphasizing the importance of proactive maintenance and adherence to strict protocols.

This detailed exploration of ALS equipment reflects only a fraction of the technological complexity inherent to modern paramedicine. The ongoing development of new technologies necessitates ongoing professional development. It's a constant process of learning and adaptation. Mastering the use of ALS equipment isn't just about technical proficiency; it's about understanding the underlying principles of patient physiology, pharmacology, and critical care. It is also about recognizing the limitations of technology and maintaining a critical and reflective approach to its application. The integration of technology in prehospital care continues to evolve, and paramedics must continuously adapt to stay abreast of the latest developments and ensure they provide the highest quality of care. The commitment to continuous learning and proficiency in utilizing advanced life support equipment is not just a professional responsibility; it's a commitment to saving lives. It's a commitment I, and every dedicated paramedic, takes seriously.

The seamless integration of advanced life support equipment into the efficient delivery of prehospital care is only half the equation. The other, equally critical, component is the safe and effective operation of the emergency vehicle itself. The ambulance, a symbol of urgent intervention, becomes a potential instrument of harm if not handled with precision, skill, and unwavering respect for the rules of the road. Many paramedics, myself included, have witnessed firsthand the devastating consequences of accidents involving emergency vehicles. These aren't just statistics; they are tragedies that irrevocably impact patients, bystanders, and the paramedics involved.

My early years in the service were marked by a naive confidence in my driving abilities. I was young, eager to prove myself, and perhaps a little too quick on the siren. I'd often find myself pushing the limits, weaving through traffic with a sense of urgency that bordered on recklessness. It wasn't until I responded to a scene where another emergency vehicle had been involved in a collision—an incident that resulted in severe injuries to the occupants of the other vehicle and a traumatic experience for the crew—that my perspective shifted fundamentally. That moment forced a deep introspection about my driving habits and the profound responsibility I carry behind the wheel.

Safe emergency vehicle operation is not simply about getting to the scene quickly; it's about arriving safely and in a condition to provide effective patient care. Speed is essential, but it's only one component of effective emergency response. The other crucial factors include defensive driving, anticipation of potential hazards, and a thorough understanding of both local and national driving regulations. The paramedic's responsibility extends beyond the immediate care of the patient; it encompasses the safety of the public, their crewmates, and themselves.

Emergency driving demands a heightened level of situational awareness. This involves constantly scanning the environment, anticipating potential hazards, and reacting proactively to prevent accidents. This is not a passive act; it necessitates active observation, anticipating the actions of other drivers, pedestrians, and cyclists. A constant mental checklist – checking mirrors, blind spots, assessing traffic flow and speed, anticipating potential hazards such as intersections, pedestrians, and construction zones – is an integral part of our daily operational routine. This is a skill honed through years of experience and continuous self-assessment. It is a practice that extends beyond the emergency response phase, influencing every aspect of ambulance operation, from routine transfers to non-emergency transports.

Defensive driving is a crucial element of safe emergency response. It means anticipating potential hazards and taking evasive actions to avoid collisions. This includes maintaining a safe following distance, even with sirens and lights activated, adapting driving techniques to different weather conditions, being prepared for sudden stops or changes in traffic flow, and always being aware that other drivers may not always yield appropriately. In heavy traffic, this means adjusting speeds and utilizing alternative routes to minimize risk, understanding that a few extra minutes saved might be an invaluable investment in safety. This strategy reduces reaction time to potential threats, allowing us the necessary room for maneuver to prevent a hazardous situation.

The legal framework governing emergency vehicle operation varies significantly across jurisdictions. Understanding these specific laws and regulations is not just a matter of compliance; it's crucial for safe and efficient operation. Knowledge of local ordinances, state regulations, and national guidelines is paramount, ensuring that we operate within the legal boundaries while still acting swiftly and effectively. This includes understanding the legal implications of siren use, right-of-way rules, and the limitations on speed and maneuverability in specific situations, ensuring we are compliant with all relevant regulations. The knowledge of these regulations is not simply a legal requirement; it is a critical factor that influences our decision-making processes.

Beyond legal requirements, certain standardized practices universally contribute to safer emergency driving. One such practice involves consistently using turn signals, even in emergency situations. This may seem counterintuitive – why alert others to our movements when urgency dictates swift actions? It's vital because it helps other drivers predict our movements and make informed decisions. Sudden, unanticipated maneuvers, especially at intersections, significantly increase the risk of a collision, even with sirens engaged. Consistently employing signals allows others to anticipate our intentions, enhancing overall safety.

Another crucial aspect of safe driving involves the importance of team communication within the ambulance. Clear and concise communication between the driver and the paramedic attending to the patient helps coordinate actions and anticipate potential hazards. Verbal cues about approaching intersections, road conditions, or unusual traffic patterns can enable the medic to prepare for changes in the vehicle's movement, optimizing patient safety and assisting with seamless care delivery. The driver needs to anticipate not only the road but also the needs of their crewmate. A simple phrase like, "Intersection approaching," can allow the medic to secure equipment, or prepare for a sudden deceleration. This effective teamwork is a cornerstone of safety.

Regular training and continuing education play a critical role in maintaining safe driving practices. Refresher courses on emergency vehicle operation should be integrated into annual professional development, focusing on techniques like defensive driving, hazard recognition, and situational awareness. Simulated emergency driving scenarios, ideally with experienced instructors providing feedback, can significantly improve reaction times and decision-making skills in high-pressure situations. These exercises help bridge the gap between theoretical knowledge and practical application, enabling better anticipation and reaction to real-world scenarios.

Technology has also played a significant role in improving emergency vehicle safety. Advanced navigation systems offer real-time traffic updates, suggesting optimal routes and minimizing response times without compromising safety. Vehicle telematics, that is, systems that record driving data like speed, braking, and acceleration, can be invaluable tools for analyzing driving patterns, identifying areas for improvement, and ensuring adherence to safe operating procedures. These technologies don't replace vigilance and skill; rather, they are valuable additions, providing enhanced situational awareness and data-driven insights that improve efficiency and safety.

Beyond the tangible aspects of emergency vehicle operation, there exists the less quantifiable yet critical element of mental and physical well-being. The demanding nature of the job, coupled with the constant exposure to stressful situations, can impact a paramedic's ability to maintain focus and make sound judgments. Fatigue, stress, and even emotional exhaustion can significantly impair driving skills. Recognizing these factors and implementing strategies to mitigate their impact is vital for the long-term safety of the paramedic and the public. Maintaining a healthy lifestyle, practicing mindfulness techniques, and seeking support when needed are not just personal benefits; they are essential aspects of safe driving practices.

In conclusion, safe and effective emergency vehicle operation is not merely a set of rules and regulations; it's a philosophy that emphasizes a commitment to safety and responsibility. It necessitates continuous learning, rigorous self-assessment, and a deep understanding of the complex interplay between speed, skill, and situational awareness. Our job is not just to respond swiftly to emergencies but to do so in a manner that safeguards the well-being of everyone involved. It's a responsibility we accept and one we continually strive to uphold, recognizing that every time we respond to a call, we are entrusted with a precious responsibility, the safe passage from point A to point B in service of others. That commitment to safety underpins all aspects of our work and, fundamentally, is what distinguishes a truly exceptional paramedic.

The ability to communicate effectively is as crucial to paramedicine as the most advanced medical equipment. Our effectiveness hinges not only on our clinical skills but also on our capacity to seamlessly integrate information, coordinate resources, and relay critical details across multiple platforms. This section explores the evolution and current state of communication technologies utilized in modern paramedicine, technologies that have become indispensable tools in our fight to save lives.

The ubiquitous two-way radio remains the cornerstone of our communication network. For decades, these devices have served as the lifeline connecting paramedics in the field with dispatch centers, hospitals, and other emergency responders. The crackle of static followed by a clear voice relaying vital information – a patient's condition, location, and needs – is a familiar sound to anyone who has worked in emergency medical services. However, the simple radio has evolved significantly. Modern radios are increasingly sophisticated, incorporating features like GPS tracking, pre-programmed messages for standardized reporting, and encrypted channels to maintain patient confidentiality. The integration of GPS allows dispatch to track our location in real-time, optimizing response times and providing critical information to responding units. Pre-programmed messages streamline communication, ensuring consistency and reducing ambiguity during crucial moments. Encrypted channels protect sensitive patient information, a critical component of maintaining patient privacy and adhering to HIPAA regulations.

Despite the advancements, radio communication presents unique challenges. The inherent limitations of radio frequency transmission, especially in urban environments or areas with geographical obstacles, can cause signal degradation or complete loss of communication. Interference from other signals, construction, or even weather patterns can disrupt transmission, creating moments of anxiety and potential delays in treatment. I remember vividly one instance where a sudden and intense thunderstorm wiped out our radio communication completely for over an hour. We were forced to rely on our own resourcefulness and limited cell service to coordinate with dispatch and the receiving hospital, an experience that underscored the limitations of even the most advanced radio systems. Such experiences reinforce the need for backup communication methods and the importance of situational awareness and adapting to unexpected challenges.

This necessity for backup communication has led to the widespread adoption of mobile data terminals (MDTs). These in-vehicle computers, typically integrated into the ambulance's dashboard, provide access to a wealth of information, including patient records, hospital bed availability, and real-time traffic data. MDTs also offer crucial data transmission capabilities, allowing paramedics to send and receive messages, transmit electrocardiograms (ECGs), and even communicate directly with hospital physicians via secure messaging systems. The ability to transmit an ECG in real-time, for example, allows physicians to assess the patient's cardiac rhythm and provide guidance on treatment before the patient even arrives at the hospital, often proving to be the difference in a time-critical situation. The value of immediate access to information, especially the ability to ascertain hospital capacity and divert to a facility better suited for the patient's needs, significantly improves patient care.

The integration of MDTs, however, isn't without its limitations. The reliance on technology introduces the potential for system failures, software glitches, or connectivity issues. A system crash in the middle of a critical response is not just an inconvenience; it can drastically reduce our ability to efficiently assess the situation and coordinate emergency care. Therefore, regular maintenance, software updates, and rigorous testing are essential to maintain the reliability of these critical systems. Furthermore, cybersecurity concerns are increasingly significant, requiring careful implementation of secure protocols to protect sensitive patient data and prevent unauthorized access.

Cellular technology has also played a transformative role in paramedic communication. Mobile phones provide a reliable backup communication system, particularly in areas with weak radio signals. The advent of smartphones with advanced features further enhances this capability. Applications specifically designed for emergency medical services provide secure messaging, real-time location tracking, and access to medical information databases. Such technology allows us to remain connected with the hospital throughout transport, providing real-time updates on the patient's condition, assisting in the preparation of the emergency department, and streamlining the process of patient handover.

Even with the array of advanced technologies, clear, concise, and effective communication remains a paramount skill that no technology can entirely replace. The ability to quickly and accurately convey complex medical information under stress is a skill honed over years of experience and rigorous training. Effective communication is not merely about transmitting information; it's about building rapport, understanding the needs of others, and ensuring that information is not only received but understood. During stressful situations, clear instructions are crucial to both patient care and overall scene safety. For instance, effective communication with bystanders can ensure scene safety, and clear communication with the patient can foster trust and cooperation.

The evolution of communication technologies in paramedicine has undoubtedly enhanced our ability to provide timely and effective care. Yet, it's essential to recognize the limitations of any technology and the crucial role of human interaction and critical thinking in ensuring successful outcomes. The integration of multiple communication platforms – radios, MDTs, cellular devices – creates a robust and redundant system, enhancing resilience and ensuring continued communication even in the face of technical difficulties. Maintaining proficiency in utilizing these technologies, coupled with a deep understanding of their limitations and an unwavering commitment to clear, concise communication, remains essential to delivering the highest quality of prehospital care.

Beyond the hardware, the development of standardized communication protocols is paramount for optimizing efficiency. Clear, concise, and consistent terminology is essential to ensuring that information is accurately and efficiently relayed between different members of the healthcare team, including emergency medical dispatchers, paramedics, hospital staff, and other emergency responders. The use of standardized reporting forms and established communication protocols reduces ambiguity, minimizes errors, and enhances overall coordination. This standardization allows seamless integration of information into the patient's record, reducing redundancies and enhancing the quality of information available throughout the patient's journey through the healthcare system.

Furthermore, the use of advanced communication technologies necessitates a high level of cybersecurity awareness and protocols. Protecting patient data from unauthorized access is not just a legal obligation; it is a moral imperative. The implementation of secure communication systems, regular software updates, and employee training on data security measures are essential to ensuring the confidentiality and integrity of patient information. This requires a continuous effort, adapting to the ever-evolving landscape of cyber threats and ensuring that our systems remain secure. The consequences of a data breach are not only devastating to the patients involved but can also have severe legal and reputational consequences for the organization.

In conclusion, communication technologies have fundamentally reshaped the landscape of paramedicine. From the simple two-way radio to the sophisticated MDTs and integrated cellular systems, technology has significantly enhanced our ability to coordinate resources, relay critical information, and provide timely and effective patient care. However, technology is merely a tool. Its effectiveness hinges on the proficiency of the users, a deep understanding of its capabilities and limitations, and an unwavering commitment to clear, concise, and effective communication, ultimately ensuring that our patients receive the best possible care. Our role remains not merely as technicians but as skilled communicators, adept at navigating the complex interplay of technology and human interaction in the relentless pursuit of saving lives.

The seamless flow of information doesn't end with dispatch and hospital communication. It continues with meticulously detailed and accurate medical documentation, a cornerstone of effective paramedicine and a critical component of patient care. This documentation serves multiple purposes, extending far beyond simply recording the events of a single call. It forms the foundation for continuous patient care, facilitates communication among healthcare providers, aids in research and quality improvement initiatives, and provides crucial legal protection for both the paramedic and the patient. The accuracy and completeness of our patient care reports are not just administrative tasks; they are vital to ensuring the best possible outcomes for those in our care.

The process begins even before we reach the patient. Before touching a patient, or even approaching the scene, it's crucial to note the time, the location, and the initial dispatch information. This initial information-gathering phase sets the stage for a complete and coherent record. I vividly recall a case where an apparent simple fall quickly escalated into something far more complex. The initial dispatch information indicated a fall, but the scene revealed underlying conditions we would not have otherwise known, leading to a different treatment plan and a faster trip to the appropriate medical facility. The initial information sets the context, a framework upon which the details of the case are built.

Once on-scene, a methodical approach to patient assessment is vital, and this must be meticulously documented. Each step of the assessment process – the patient's initial presentation, vital signs, physical examination findings, and any interventions performed – should be clearly and concisely recorded. This record needs to be comprehensive, covering not only obvious injuries but also potential underlying conditions. A simple laceration might be indicative of a more serious underlying problem, for example, a seemingly isolated injury could suggest domestic abuse, a point that must be carefully considered and documented.

Observing subtle clues can be crucial in painting a complete picture of the patient's condition.

The use of standardized terminology and abbreviations is crucial. A standardized language ensures clarity and minimizes the potential for misinterpretations. Using medical terminology correctly is essential; however, using excessively obscure terms, or acronyms not universally understood, can lead to ambiguities that hinder the seamless transmission of critical information to colleagues and other healthcare providers. Clear, precise language, devoid of jargon, ensures everyone involved understands the patient's condition and the actions taken. For example, instead of using overly technical terms, writing "patient is unresponsive" instead of "patient exhibits an absence of spontaneous motor activity" is preferable.

Beyond the immediate clinical findings, the documentation should include a narrative description of the entire event. This narrative provides context, explaining the circumstances surrounding the incident, the interventions performed, and the patient's response to treatment. It includes crucial details like the patient's level of consciousness, their responsiveness to stimuli, and the sequence of events leading up to the emergency call. Moreover, this part of the documentation allows for an account of any challenges encountered at the scene – environmental hazards, difficulties in accessing the patient, or any obstacles that hampered the delivery of care. I once responded to a call in a dense wooded area, where navigating the terrain was extremely challenging. The details of this navigation were not only important for the incident report, but also contributed to an internal review of our response procedures for similar incidents.

Furthermore, the documentation must include the details of the treatment provided. This includes the medications administered, the dosages, and the routes of administration. All procedures performed should be documented with precision, including the rationale behind each intervention. For example, while administering oxygen, noting the patient's oxygen saturation before and after administration, as well as their respiratory rate, helps us demonstrate the effectiveness of the intervention, providing critical information for the receiving hospital and ensuring the patient receives optimal treatment. The lack of this detail could lead to significant issues in patient care during transitions.

The patient's response to treatment must also be meticulously documented. This involves recording any changes in the patient's condition, both positive and negative, as well as any adverse reactions to the medications or procedures. The evolution of the patient's status is critical, showing the effectiveness of our interventions and providing valuable information to the receiving hospital. For example, noting a decrease in pain level or an improvement in respiratory rate demonstrates the positive impact of our actions, offering the hospital staff valuable insights into the patient's progress. Failure to adequately document these changes undermines the continuity of care.

Beyond the clinical details, the documentation should also capture the patient's response to the intervention provided, highlighting the patient's condition after treatment. Furthermore, this is where the patient's family interactions, particularly their consent and refusal of treatments, and their overall emotional state should be carefully recorded. Their responses should be noted accurately, contributing to the patient's overall medical history.

The completion of the patient care report is not merely a clerical task; it's a vital part of the patient care continuum. The information gathered in this report provides the receiving hospital with essential information for continuing treatment. Clear, concise, and accurate documentation enables a smooth transition of care, minimizing delays and potential errors. Furthermore, our patient reports play a key role in ensuring efficient use of resources. In case of medicolegal issues, the quality of documentation serves as a legal defense and acts as a reliable record of the events and actions that transpired during the emergency call.

Furthermore, thorough documentation assists in quality improvement initiatives. By analyzing trends and patterns identified in patient care reports, we can improve our response strategies, refine our treatment protocols, and identify areas requiring further training or resource allocation. This continuous cycle of evaluation and improvement is essential to enhancing the quality of prehospital care.

Accurate and efficient record-keeping is also crucial for legal and regulatory compliance. Patient confidentiality must be strictly maintained, adhering to HIPAA regulations and any other relevant local or state laws. Incomplete, inaccurate, or poorly written documentation can have serious legal implications, so precision and adherence to protocols are absolutely paramount.

Finally, effective documentation is essential for personal professional development. Reviewing our own patient care reports allows us to reflect on our performance, identify areas for improvement, and enhance our clinical skills. It provides a mechanism for continuous learning, encouraging self-reflection and improvement in our approach to patient care. Regular review of past reports provides not only a historical record, but also allows for the identification of trends and patterns, enabling better preparation and response to future incidents. Therefore, reflective practice, driven by reviewing the quality of documentation, acts as a mechanism for growth and enhancement in paramedicine practice.

In conclusion, medical documentation is far more than just a bureaucratic requirement; it's a vital tool that supports high-quality patient care, facilitates interprofessional communication, enables continuous quality improvement, protects both paramedics and patients, and assists in legal compliance. Mastering the art of accurate and efficient medical record-keeping is an ongoing process, demanding a commitment to detail, clarity, and a thorough understanding of the legal and ethical considerations involved. It's a skill honed through experience and a reflection of our dedication to providing the best possible care in every situation, every time.

The evolution of paramedicine is inextricably linked to technological advancements. What was once a field reliant on basic tools and intuition is rapidly transforming into a technologically sophisticated profession. This transformation is driven by a desire to improve patient outcomes, enhance efficiency, and address the ever-increasing demands placed upon emergency medical services (EMS). The future of paramedicine is not just about faster ambulances; it's about leveraging technology to provide more accurate diagnoses, administer more effective treatments, and ultimately, save more lives.

One of the most significant shifts is the burgeoning field of telehealth. Imagine a scenario where a paramedic, on scene with a patient experiencing chest pain, can instantly transmit an electrocardiogram (ECG) to a cardiologist at a remote hospital. The cardiologist can then review the data in real-time, offering immediate guidance on the most appropriate course of action. This isn't science fiction; it's the reality shaping the future of paramedicine. Telehealth allows for remote consultations with specialists, providing immediate expert advice in situations where seconds matter.

This is particularly valuable in rural or underserved areas where access to specialists may be limited, bridging the geographical gap in healthcare access. The speed and efficiency of this communication can drastically shorten decision-making times, potentially saving lives and improving patient outcomes. I recall a case where a patient exhibiting symptoms of a stroke was far from a major hospital. Through telehealth consultation with a neurologist, we were able to implement a faster treatment protocol, initiating the correct medication before even reaching the hospital—a scenario unimaginable just a few years ago.

Telehealth isn't limited to ECG transmissions. Advances in mobile technology and broadband connectivity are enabling the transmission of high-resolution images and videos, allowing remote specialists to visually assess injuries, monitor vital signs, and provide guidance on procedures. Furthermore, the capacity to transmit patient data, including medical history and medication lists, directly to the receiving hospital ensures a seamless transfer of care, minimizing potential communication errors and delays. The integration of wearable sensors and remote monitoring devices further enhances the possibilities of telehealth, enabling continuous monitoring of vital signs even after the patient has been discharged from the hospital. This could significantly decrease hospital readmissions and allow for earlier interventions in case of complications.

The integration of artificial intelligence (AI) is another transformative force reshaping paramedicine. AI algorithms can analyze vast amounts of data—from patient vital signs to medical history and geographical location—to predict the likelihood of adverse events, identify potential diagnoses, and optimize treatment strategies. AI-powered diagnostic tools can assist paramedics in identifying subtle signs and symptoms that might be missed by the human eye, leading to earlier and more accurate diagnoses. For instance, an AI-powered system could analyze an ECG more quickly and effectively than a human, potentially detecting subtle arrhythmias that might otherwise go unnoticed, leading to more timely interventions.

While AI holds immense promise, its integration into paramedicine also raises ethical considerations. Concerns about data privacy and security, algorithm bias, and the potential for over-reliance on technology need careful consideration and robust safeguards. The potential for algorithmic bias to influence treatment decisions based on demographic factors needs to be addressed proactively. Transparency and accountability in the development and deployment of AI tools are essential to ensure equitable and ethical care for all patients. The human element remains crucial. AI should be viewed as a powerful tool to augment, not replace, the expertise and judgment of experienced paramedics.

Remote diagnostics, powered by AI and sophisticated sensing technology, are poised to further revolutionize prehospital care. Imagine a scenario where a paramedic equipped with a portable ultrasound device can conduct a rapid assessment of a patient's internal organs, transmitting the images for real-time analysis by a radiologist. This could dramatically improve the accuracy and speed of diagnoses in critical situations, informing immediate treatment decisions and improving patient outcomes. These technologies are still developing, but their potential to transform paramedicine is enormous. Consider a scenario where a paramedic is faced with a trauma patient in a remote location. The ability to conduct point-of-care testing, analyze blood samples for crucial information, and transmit this information to a hospital before even reaching the facility can completely redefine the scope of care in rural and remote areas.

Beyond the aforementioned technologies, advancements in other areas will continue to impact paramedicine. Improved materials for emergency vehicles, more sophisticated life support equipment, and advancements in drug delivery systems will all contribute to enhanced patient care. The development of more effective and safer medications will continue to improve treatment options. Research into regenerative medicine and other advanced therapies could lead to breakthroughs that redefine how we manage trauma and critical illnesses. The use of augmented reality (AR) could revolutionize training and education.

However, the integration of advanced technologies into paramedicine isn't without its challenges. The costs associated with acquiring and maintaining these technologies can be substantial, potentially creating disparities in access between well-resourced and under-resourced EMS agencies. Furthermore, the need for ongoing training and professional development to keep pace with rapid technological advancements is crucial. Paramedics will need to develop a high level of technological literacy to effectively utilize these tools and ensure patient safety. And the potential for technology malfunctions or cyberattacks adds another layer of complexity. Robust cybersecurity measures and effective backup systems are crucial to prevent disruption of service and protect patient data.

The future of paramedicine will undoubtedly be shaped by ongoing innovation and technological advancements. The ethical considerations, cost implications, and necessary training requirements for the adoption of these innovations all require careful and thoughtful consideration. But the potential benefits—improved patient outcomes, increased efficiency, and expanded access to care—make the pursuit of these advancements a critical imperative for the future of the profession. Embracing these technologies responsibly and strategically will help us to continue providing the highest quality of care to those who need it most. The path forward requires a balance between embracing the transformative power of technology and maintaining the fundamental human connection at the heart of paramedicine, ensuring that even with the most advanced tools, we never lose sight of the individual human being facing an emergency.

6

The Human Element: Patient Interaction

B uilding rapport, that unspoken connection forged in the crucible of crisis, is arguably the most crucial skill a paramedic can possess. It's not just about administering medication or applying splints; it's about navigating the emotional landscape of a terrifying situation, offering solace and understanding amidst chaos. This ability to connect, to truly *see* the patient beyond their injuries, is what transforms a skilled technician into a compassionate caregiver. It's what allows us to effectively manage not only the physical but also the psychological aspects of an emergency.

I recall a particularly vivid call involving a young woman who had fallen from a significant height. The scene was chaotic: flashing lights, sirens, a crowd of onlookers. Her injuries were severe, and the pain was evident in her every strained breath. But what struck me most was the overwhelming fear in her eyes, the palpable terror that overshadowed the physical agony. My initial assessment focused on her injuries, of course, but my priority quickly shifted to calming her fear. I spoke softly, explaining each step of the procedure in simple terms, answering her questions patiently, even when they were repetitive. I focused on making eye contact, offering a reassuring smile, and allowing her to hold my hand. It wasn't a dramatic intervention, no heroic act, but it was crucial. It humanized the situation, turning the sterile clinical environment into a space of empathy and shared understanding. The successful stabilization of her condition paled in comparison to the quiet comfort I managed to bring to her in those initial moments.

Effective communication is the cornerstone of rapport building. It's not simply about delivering information; it's about truly listening, understanding the patient's perspective, and validating their feelings. Active listening, a technique often emphasized in paramedic training, involves more than just hearing words; it requires paying attention to nonverbal cues like body language and tone of voice. It demands empathy. Imagine a patient experiencing chest pain, their words laced with fear and uncertainty. Simply responding with, "Your vitals are stable," offers minimal reassurance. A more effective approach might be, "I understand you're feeling scared. Your heart rate is elevated, but we're going to work together to make sure you're alright." This response acknowledges the patient's emotional state, creating a space for trust and collaboration. By using words that mirror the patient's emotional state, we reflect their inner world, making them feel seen and understood. This often reduces anxiety levels, which in turn allows for more effective communication and potentially better patient cooperation.

Active listening extends beyond verbal communication. Nonverbal cues are essential. Maintaining eye contact demonstrates attentiveness and respect. A gentle touch, if appropriate and culturally sensitive, can offer comfort and reassurance. It is important to be mindful of cultural differences; a touch considered comforting in one culture might be perceived as intrusive in another. Our awareness of this variation is critical in building trust. I once responded to a call involving an elderly gentleman from a different culture who was hesitant to engage with me. He felt more comfortable talking once I simply offered him a quiet presence and a respectful distance. Building trust took time and genuine effort, but this quiet, respectful observation ultimately proved far more effective than any rushed attempt at physical examination.

The importance of active listening extends to families as well. Often, families are equally, if not more, distressed than the patient themselves. They witness the suddenness of the crisis, the vulnerability of their loved one, and feel the overwhelming fear of the unknown. They need reassurance, information, and empathy just as much as the patient. Imagine the fear a parent feels watching paramedics work on their child, or the anguish of a spouse seeing their partner struggling to breathe. Providing updates regularly, explaining procedures in lay terms, and answering their questions honestly (within the limits of our medical knowledge) are vital. Being able to say "I understand this is terrifying for you" or "I know you're worried, but we're doing everything we can," goes a long way in diffusing anxiety. Often, these moments of connection, the acknowledgment of their emotional turmoil, are more impactful than any medical intervention. It is not always possible to provide a definitive answer in the middle of an urgent situation, but offering comfort and acknowledging their concerns is paramount.

However, building rapport is not always straightforward. Some patients, understandably, are hesitant to trust us, particularly if they have had negative experiences with the healthcare system in the past. Others may be in such distress or disorientation that communication is difficult. In such cases, patience and a non-judgmental approach are crucial. We might need to try different communication strategies, perhaps using simplified language or focusing on nonverbal cues. A calm demeanor, a gentle voice, and a reassuring presence can often ease anxiety even when a coherent conversation is not immediately possible.

Another aspect of rapport-building lies in effective use of therapeutic communication techniques. This involves creating a safe space for expression, allowing the patient and family to articulate their fears, concerns, and experiences. It often requires the paramedic to use empathy and reflection to make sure they have truly heard and understood. Using phrases like, "That sounds really difficult," or, "It makes sense you'd feel that way," validate their feelings without dismissing or minimizing their pain. Moreover, using reflective questioning techniques – repeating what the patient says in their own words – can help to clarify their needs and concerns. It helps to build a rapport of trust because it affirms that they have been heard.

Furthermore, a paramedic must be self-aware and manage their own emotions effectively. Stress, fatigue, and the emotional toll of the job can easily impact our ability to connect with patients. If we are overwhelmed by our own emotions, our ability to empathize with others is diminished. Self-care, including adequate rest, healthy lifestyle choices, and seeking support when needed, are therefore non-negotiable for any paramedic who wishes to maintain effective rapport-building skills. Practicing mindfulness or other stress-management techniques can help to manage our own emotional responses and improve our ability to stay grounded and present in challenging situations.

Finally, the most critical element is empathy—the ability to understand and share the feelings of another. It's not about feeling *what* the patient feels but *understanding* what they are feeling. This profound understanding allows us to respond in a way that meets their emotional needs as well as their medical ones. It's the difference between seeing a broken leg and seeing a person enduring immense pain and fear because of it. And it's this empathy that helps us connect, to build rapport, and to provide the best possible care, not just medically, but humanely. The most profound moments in my career haven't been defined by the technical aspects of the job but by the quiet moments of human connection, the unspoken understanding shared in the midst of chaos. It is a connection that heals, soothes, and often, saves. And that, more than anything, defines what it means to be a truly effective paramedic.

Our ability to connect with patients, as previously discussed, forms the bedrock of effective paramedicine. However, this connection transcends simply understanding the immediate medical needs; it necessitates a deep understanding of the cultural context surrounding each patient. Cultural competency, the ability to interact effectively with people from diverse cultural backgrounds, is not merely a desirable trait; it's a fundamental requirement for providing truly equitable and compassionate care. Ignoring cultural differences can lead to miscommunication, mistrust, and ultimately, suboptimal treatment.

One striking example that comes to mind involves a call to a residence within a predominantly Hmong community. We responded to a report of a woman experiencing severe abdominal pain. While my partner expertly conducted a physical assessment, I attempted to communicate with the patient, who spoke very little English. Initially, I relied heavily on basic phrases and gestures, but I quickly realized my approach was inadequate. Her discomfort wasn't solely physical; it was evident in her withdrawn demeanor and anxious glances towards her family members. They, too, appeared hesitant to engage fully.

My initial attempts at communication felt sterile, almost invasive. My medical training focused on symptoms and treatment protocols, not on understanding the nuances of cultural communication. I realized my failure to create a space where she felt safe and respected—a space where her cultural background would be acknowledged and respected—was hindering my ability to provide adequate care. The family's apprehension stemmed, I later learned, from a deep-rooted distrust of Western medicine, a mistrust fueled by past experiences and cultural beliefs. They preferred to trust traditional healing methods first.

Fortunately, we had a colleague who was fluent in Hmong. Her presence transformed the situation. Through her, we learned that the patient's pain wasn't just physical; it involved deeply held cultural beliefs about illness and healing. Her reluctance wasn't disobedience; it was a manifestation of her cultural background. Understanding this drastically altered our approach. We didn't dismiss her preferences but instead sought to integrate them with our medical expertise. We explained our intentions respectfully, highlighting the potential benefits of Western medical intervention while assuring them we wouldn't disregard their traditional practices. With this bridge of understanding built, the patient's trust grew, and the subsequent examination and treatment became significantly more efficient and effective. The success of this intervention wasn't in a specific procedure but in demonstrating cultural sensitivity and respect.

This experience underscored a critical lesson: cultural competency is not a checklist to be completed; it's an ongoing process of learning and adapting. It demands continuous education, a willingness to acknowledge our own biases, and an unwavering commitment to understanding diverse perspectives. In our multicultural society, patients come from a variety of religious, spiritual, and cultural backgrounds. Their beliefs and practices can significantly influence their interactions with the healthcare system. Some cultures may favor a holistic approach to healing that integrates physical, mental, and spiritual well-being. Others might hold strong religious beliefs that may influence their medical decisions, such as the refusal of blood transfusions or specific treatments.

Understanding a patient's religious beliefs is often crucial in their care. For example, a patient from a certain religious background might observe certain dietary restrictions which need to be considered when providing them with food or hydration. Similarly, a patient might have specific beliefs about the afterlife or end-of-life care. Respecting these beliefs is not merely a matter of politeness but a critical aspect of providing humane and holistic care. Ignoring them can lead to mistrust and even conflict. The goal isn't to force a patient to abandon their beliefs but to incorporate them into their treatment plan, creating a framework that respects their faith while maintaining medical efficacy.

Cultural competency extends beyond religious and spiritual beliefs. It also encompasses understanding a patient's family dynamics and social support networks. In many cultures, family members play a central role in decision-making and healthcare. Disregarding this fundamental aspect of their culture might be perceived as disrespectful and lead to distrust. For instance, in some families, it might be customary for the eldest male family member to make medical decisions on behalf of the patient, regardless of the patient's own preferences. Ignoring this familial hierarchy could result in a breakdown of communication and hinder the treatment process. Therefore, we must strive to include family members in the discussion whenever appropriate, ensuring their participation is both meaningful and respectful.

Furthermore, cultural sensitivity dictates a clear understanding of nonverbal communication. What might be deemed acceptable behavior in one culture could be considered deeply offensive in another. Eye contact, physical touch, and personal space are all subject to considerable cultural variation. Direct eye contact, for instance, is interpreted differently across various cultures. In some cultures, it signifies respect and attentiveness; in others, it might be considered rude or challenging. Similarly, the idea of personal space varies. What one person considers a comfortable distance may be seen as invasive by another. Such variances necessitate careful observation and an awareness of the potential for misinterpretation.

It is crucial to be mindful of the language barrier in providing care. While proficiency in multiple languages is an invaluable asset, effective communication can often be achieved through creative problem-solving, utilizing tools such as translation apps, bilingual dictionaries, or even relying on visual aids. Never underestimate the power of simple, clear communication. When using interpreters, it's crucial to address our message directly to the patient and not solely to the interpreter.

This shows respect and ensures that the patient feels engaged and understood.

Moreover, we must recognize that healthcare experiences can be profoundly affected by socioeconomic factors. Patients from lower socioeconomic backgrounds might face unique challenges in accessing care, including financial constraints, limited transportation options, and lower levels of health literacy. Addressing these concerns requires a compassionate and understanding approach. This might entail assisting them with resources such as transportation assistance, explaining complicated medical terms in plain language, or connecting them with community services that can alleviate their financial burdens. Our goal is to provide high-quality care that is not hindered by external factors.

Cultural competency is not a one-size-fits-all approach. It's a complex and multifaceted issue that demands ongoing education and self-reflection. Regular training on cultural sensitivity is essential for all paramedics. This training should not only include theoretical learning but also hands-on practice through role-playing scenarios and simulations. This will allow for refinement and improvements in their approach. Continuous learning must also involve personal reflections on experiences with diverse patient populations, identifying areas for improvement and fostering a culture of respectful dialogue. Building these skills needs to be an ongoing commitment, not a one-time exercise.

The development of cultural competency also requires us to create an environment of openness and curiosity. We need to be comfortable asking questions about a patient's background, beliefs, and preferences. These questions must be posed with sincerity and respect, always ensuring the patient feels comfortable sharing or not sharing personal information. In these discussions, it's essential to approach each patient as an individual, respecting their unique experiences and circumstances, while avoiding making generalizations or stereotypes.

Ultimately, providing culturally competent care enhances the overall quality of paramedic services. It fosters trust, improves communication, and leads to more effective interventions. It isn't simply about adhering to a set of guidelines; it's about embracing a philosophy of empathy, respect, and understanding. It's about recognizing that each patient, regardless of their background, deserves to be treated with dignity and compassion. It's about approaching each call with the awareness that we are not just treating an illness, but a person—a person wrapped in a rich tapestry of cultural experiences, beliefs, and practices. And it's this holistic understanding that elevates us from skilled technicians to compassionate caregivers, capable of delivering not just effective medical care but genuinely humane service. The ultimate measure of our success isn't just in saving lives but in doing so with a profound sensitivity and respect for each patient's unique identity and cultural context.

Breaking bad news is arguably one of the most challenging aspects of paramedicine. It's a skill honed not just through training, but through experience, empathy, and a deep understanding of human nature. The technical proficiency required to stabilize a patient is undeniably crucial, but the emotional intelligence needed to deliver devastating news with grace and compassion is equally, if not more, vital. It's a moment where our role transcends the purely medical; we become a conduit of support, a source of comfort amidst unimaginable pain.

I remember a call vividly, one that still resonates with me years later. We responded to a multi-vehicle accident on a rain-slicked highway. Amidst the chaos, we found a young woman trapped in her vehicle, her injuries severe. Despite our best efforts, it was clear from the outset that her condition was critical. While my partner attended to her immediate physical needs, I began assessing her mental state, trying to build a connection amidst the wreckage. Her eyes, though filled with pain, held a glimmer of hope, a desperate clinging to life.

The doctor at the scene, after a thorough assessment, made the decision to airlift her to a trauma center. While arranging transport, he turned to me and, with a somber shake of his head, indicated that despite the best efforts, survival was unlikely. It fell to me to break this devastating news to her distraught mother, who had arrived at the scene, her face a mask of anxiety and anticipation.

My initial instinct was to avoid the truth, to cushion the blow with vague reassurances. But years of experience, and the memory of countless difficult conversations, taught me the futility of such attempts. Honesty, even in its harshness, was the most compassionate approach. I began by acknowledging her obvious distress, mirroring her emotions with a gentle tone and empathetic eye contact. "I can see how worried you are," I said, choosing my words carefully, "and I want to assure you we're doing everything we can."

Then, in the simplest terms possible, I shared the prognosis, avoiding medical jargon. "The doctor believes her injuries are very severe," I explained, "and despite our best efforts, the chances of her recovery are unfortunately very slim." I paused, allowing the gravity of my words to settle, observing her reaction carefully. Her grief was immediate and visceral, a wave of sobs that shook her body. I offered her my hand, a silent gesture of support, allowing her to release her emotions without interruption.

There was no easy way to make the situation better, no magic words that could erase the pain. My job was to support her during this harrowing experience, offering her my unwavering presence. The situation itself, a devastating loss, was far more profound than any single communication. I listened, offering comforting words, but mostly focusing on acknowledging the depth of her loss, not trying to diminish or fix it. The task wasn't to mitigate her pain but to share it, to bear witness to it with compassion. It was a lesson that underscored the importance of patience, empathy, and acknowledging the limits of what we can offer as paramedics. Sometimes, our role is less about fixing problems and more about providing a much-needed shoulder to lean on amidst tragedy.

The approach to breaking bad news involves meticulous preparation. It's crucial to gather all the necessary information beforehand, ensuring a clear understanding of the patient's condition and prognosis. This minimizes any potential for ambiguity and confusion. Choosing the right setting is equally important. A private and quiet environment minimizes distractions and allows for a more intimate and sensitive conversation. It's imperative that patients are treated with respect and given time to process the information. Sometimes, the presence of loved ones can offer support and emotional fortitude, but it also necessitates navigating the dynamics of the family unit.

The delivery itself should be direct, clear, and concise. Avoid medical jargon and technical terminology; instead, use simple, straightforward language easily understood by the recipient. Start by acknowledging the emotions of the patient and their family. It's crucial to validate their feelings, showing that you understand their pain and acknowledging the impact of the bad news. Avoid false hope; honesty, however difficult, is the most compassionate approach.

After conveying the information, allow for a period of silence. Let the gravity of the situation settle, and allow the recipient to process their feelings. Be prepared for a wide range of emotional responses, from tears and anger to shock and disbelief. Your role is not to judge or control their response but to provide support and a safe space for them to express their emotions. Active listening is paramount – paying attention not only to the words spoken but also to the unspoken emotions, the nuances in their body language.

It is also imperative to offer practical assistance. Connect patients and their families with necessary resources – support groups, grief counseling, social workers. Follow-up calls can offer continued support and demonstrate ongoing care. Breaking bad news is not a one-time event; it's an ongoing process that requires continued attention and sensitivity. It demands a profound understanding of human resilience, the ability to recognize the strength within even in the face of unimaginable loss.

In my years as a paramedic, I've learned that empathy is not simply a soft skill; it's a cornerstone of effective patient care. It's not about suppressing our own emotions, but about developing the ability to understand and share the feelings of others. It's about creating a space where patients feel heard, understood, and respected, even in the most challenging circumstances. It's about recognizing that beyond the physical injuries, there's a human being grappling with fear, grief, or uncertainty. Our ability to connect with patients on this human level, to acknowledge their pain and offer support, is what transforms us from medical professionals into truly compassionate caregivers.

This holistic approach extends beyond immediate patient care. It necessitates a comprehensive understanding of the social and environmental factors that influence a patient's well-being. Socioeconomic disparities, access to healthcare, and the availability of social support networks all contribute to a patient's overall resilience and capacity to cope with adversity. A truly compassionate approach considers these broader contexts, striving to offer not just immediate medical intervention but also long-term support and guidance.

For example, a patient facing a life-altering diagnosis may also be grappling with financial insecurity or lack of access to adequate healthcare resources. In such cases, our role extends beyond simply delivering the bad news; it includes connecting the patient with social workers, financial aid programs, and other support systems that can help them navigate this difficult phase of their lives. This holistic approach, which integrates medical expertise with social responsibility, underscores the ethical imperative of compassionate care. It recognizes that providing effective medical treatment is only one aspect of a much larger equation. A complete approach considers the emotional, psychological, and social well-being of the patient, recognizing the interconnectedness of their physical and mental health.

The emotional toll of consistently delivering difficult news cannot be underestimated. Witnessing the raw grief and despair of patients and their families takes a profound emotional toll. It's crucial for paramedics to develop healthy coping mechanisms to manage this stress. This might involve regular debriefings with colleagues, seeking supervision from mental health professionals, or participating in support groups specifically designed for first responders. The ongoing self-care practices are not a sign of weakness but a testament to the resilience required to navigate the emotionally demanding aspects of the profession. Recognizing the limits of our capacity for emotional support and seeking professional help when needed is a critical component of maintaining our own well-being. This, in turn, allows us to maintain a high level of emotional intelligence, enabling us to better support our patients during their moments of crisis.

In conclusion, breaking bad news is a multifaceted skill honed through experience, empathy, and ongoing self-reflection. It necessitates direct and clear communication, active listening, and a profound understanding of human emotion. Beyond the medical aspects, it necessitates connecting patients with the necessary resources and supports. It demands a commitment to not only providing effective medical care but also offering a supportive and compassionate presence during moments of profound distress. The emotional toll of this work is significant, and ongoing self-care is critical to maintaining resilience and ensuring that paramedics can continue to offer high-quality, compassionate care. The ability to deliver difficult news with grace and compassion is a testament to our dedication as paramedics, a critical skill that transcends medical expertise and exemplifies the human element at the heart of our profession.

Managing challenging patients is an unavoidable aspect of paramedicine. It's a reality that extends far beyond the textbook scenarios we practice during training. The adrenaline-fueled urgency of a cardiac arrest is often easier to manage than the simmering tension of a patient refusing treatment, or the outright hostility of a person in crisis. These encounters require a different skillset, one rooted in de-escalation, conflict resolution, and a profound understanding of human behavior under stress. It's a skill honed not only through formal training but through the crucible of real-world experience.

One of the most valuable tools in my paramedic arsenal is the ability to actively listen. It's more than just hearing the words; it's about observing body language, recognizing nonverbal cues, and understanding the underlying emotions driving the patient's behavior. A seemingly simple complaint of chest pain might mask underlying anxiety, fear, or even anger. A patient who is verbally abusive may be reacting to an underlying fear of the unknown or a past traumatic experience. Active listening provides a window into their perspective, enabling us to respond appropriately.

For instance, I recall responding to a call for a man who had fallen and was complaining of severe back pain. He was immediately agitated, shouting and refusing our help. Instead of immediately attempting to physically assist him, which would likely have escalated the situation, I began by sitting down beside him, maintaining a calm and respectful demeanor. I offered him water and simply listened as he vented his frustration, his anger, and his fear of further injury. He wasn't just angry about his pain; he was afraid, insecure, and feeling completely out of control. Once he felt heard, his aggression gradually subsided. He expressed his fear of hospitals, a fear rooted in past negative experiences, and, importantly, his trust that I was there to help. It became a collaborative process, where his fears were addressed and he felt empowered to participate in his own care. By validating his feelings and acknowledging his fears, I managed to create a safe space for him to express his concerns without feeling further threatened.

De-escalation techniques are essential for navigating these challenging situations. Creating a safe and comfortable environment is paramount. This means maintaining a calm and non-threatening physical posture – avoiding any actions that could be interpreted as aggressive. Our tone of voice plays a vital role; a soft, empathetic tone is crucial, even when faced with hostility. Our body language should mirror calmness; maintaining eye contact (without staring intensely), while avoiding aggressive or defensive postures.

Verbal de-escalation involves a range of techniques, starting with empathy and validation. Acknowledging the patient's feelings – even if we don't agree with their behavior – is a powerful de-escalation technique. Phrases like, "I understand you're feeling frustrated right now," or "I can see you're in a lot of pain," can significantly diffuse tension. It's a reminder that we are there to care for them, even when their behavior is challenging.

Clear and concise communication is essential. Avoiding jargon and using simple, straightforward language is crucial. Repeating the patient's concerns back to them, reflecting back their emotions and summarising, is an effective way to show understanding and to ensure that we're both on the same page. This validation process allows them to feel heard and understood, reducing the anxiety that may be fueling their difficult behavior.

However, de-escalation techniques are not always enough. In some situations, conflict might escalate despite our best efforts. In these instances, having a well-defined plan for conflict resolution is vital. This plan may involve additional personnel, or securing the environment to ensure the safety of both the patient and the team. It's crucial to have a clear understanding of our limitations; knowing when to ask for backup or when a more forceful approach might be necessary is vital. This requires careful consideration and judgment that takes into account the safety of all involved.

Maintaining professional composure is paramount throughout these encounters. Remaining calm and avoiding engaging in argumentative exchanges helps to create a more supportive environment. This is sometimes very challenging; the frustration and aggression of a patient can be emotionally draining. It is in these times when active self-care and strong emotional boundaries become vital to preventing burnout and protecting our own mental health.

Self-care isn't a luxury; it's a necessity in this profession. Regular debriefings with colleagues, the opportunity to share our experiences and gain support from trusted individuals who understand our challenges is essential. Seeking professional supervision, either through counseling or other mental health support, can provide essential tools for managing the cumulative effects of consistently dealing with stress, negativity and challenging individuals.

Another crucial element in managing difficult patients is understanding their underlying needs. A patient's behavior is often a manifestation of unmet needs – whether it's physical pain, emotional distress, or a lack of information. Addressing these underlying needs can significantly de-escalate the situation. Offering pain relief, providing clear explanations, and ensuring that their questions are answered can significantly reduce the patient's agitation and hostility.

For instance, I once responded to a call for a confused and agitated elderly woman who was refusing to go to the hospital. She was visibly distressed and resistant to our care. We initially encountered significant resistance. However, by calmly assessing her situation and discovering that she was experiencing significant fear and disorientation due to delirium, we were able to address the immediate issue. We reassured her, clarified the situation, and explained the reason for our visit, all while gently calming her fears.

This involved patiently explaining the benefits of treatment, and listening to her concerns and apprehensions. We reassured her about her safety and well-being. By understanding and addressing the underlying cause of her agitation – her fear and disorientation – we were able to help her accept transport to the hospital.

Our role as paramedics often extends beyond immediate medical care. It includes providing emotional support, offering reassurance, and empowering patients to participate in their own care. This holistic approach acknowledges that medical emergencies aren't always just about physical injuries; they frequently involve complex emotional and psychological dynamics.

Effective patient interaction is not merely a soft skill; it's a fundamental component of providing high-quality paramedic care. It's a skill that requires ongoing learning, self-reflection, and a commitment to understanding human behavior under stress. It's about developing the ability to connect with patients on a human level, to acknowledge their fears, and to provide compassionate support, even in the most challenging circumstances. It's about remembering that behind the difficult behavior, there is often a person in need of help, someone struggling to cope with fear, pain, or frustration. Our ability to connect with them on this human level transforms us from medical professionals into compassionate caregivers. It's about recognizing our role extends beyond the immediate emergency and encompasses the human element, recognizing the need to validate emotional response and acknowledge the patient's perspective before focusing on the medical intervention. This understanding forms the foundation for building trust and for successfully navigating the challenges inherent in caring for difficult patients. It is, ultimately, the foundation of effective and compassionate care.

Beyond the immediate emergency, a crucial aspect of our role as paramedics is advocating for our patients. This involves ensuring they receive the quality of care they deserve and understanding their rights within the often-complex healthcare system. This advocacy goes far beyond simply administering treatment; it's about navigating bureaucratic hurdles, communicating effectively with hospital staff, and ensuring a smooth transition from our care to the next stage of their treatment. This often involves challenging systems, and sometimes even battling institutional inertia, all while keeping the patient's best interests at the forefront.

One particularly poignant instance involved a young woman, Sarah (all identifying information changed to maintain patient privacy), who sustained multiple injuries in a car accident. While her physical wounds were severe, requiring immediate surgical intervention, her insurance coverage was proving problematic. The hospital's billing department was initially hesitant to admit her without assurances of payment, a situation that brought a chilling sense of pragmatism into a critical care setting. The urgency of her situation demanded immediate action; time was literally a factor in her recovery. My years of experience taught me that delays in care can lead to complications and, in some cases, dire outcomes. I immediately contacted the hospital's social worker, explaining the urgency of Sarah's case and advocating for her admittance based on the criticality of her condition. We then moved to secure emergency authorization.

The paperwork felt overwhelming in that tense environment, but I knew that bureaucratic shortcuts often meant cutting corners when it comes to a patient's rights. After extensive phone calls, navigating confusing insurance guidelines and appealing to the hospital's ethical obligations, we finally secured authorization. While the system proved cumbersome, the relief in securing immediate care for Sarah was immense. This experience underscored the importance of patient advocacy, not merely as a professional responsibility but as a moral imperative. It showed me just how intertwined a paramedic's role is with ensuring access to timely, adequate care.

Another crucial element of patient advocacy involves understanding and explaining patients' rights. Many individuals, particularly those in vulnerable situations, might not fully understand their rights regarding healthcare decisions, consent procedures, and access to information. This is often amplified in stressful emergency situations. It's our duty to ensure that patients are informed about their options, their ability to refuse treatment (if appropriate), and their right to have a say in their medical journey. This requires patience and clear communication, especially when dealing with individuals who are experiencing pain, trauma, or confusion.

I remember responding to a call for an elderly gentleman, Mr. Jones, who was experiencing a severe asthma attack. He was visibly distressed and struggling to breathe. While providing immediate respiratory support, I noticed his reluctance to be transported to the hospital. He expressed concerns about the costs and the inconvenience. He was worried about leaving his beloved pet cat alone at home. Instead of simply focusing on the immediate medical intervention, I took the time to listen to his concerns, addressing his anxieties about the cost of hospital care. I explained his rights to access healthcare, the potential financial assistance programs, and the options available for caring for his cat during his hospital stay. After listening to his fears, I offered him a list of local pet-sitting services, and reassured him that his financial worries would be addressed.

The simple act of acknowledging his concerns and helping him find practical solutions transformed the situation. Mr. Jones, relieved and confident that his needs were understood and addressed, willingly accepted transport to the hospital. This small act of advocacy, beyond the immediate medical need, demonstrated the power of understanding the patient's circumstances and addressing concerns well beyond the confines of immediate medical intervention.

Sometimes, advocacy involves challenging healthcare professionals and systems. While the vast majority of doctors and nurses share our commitment to patient well-being, there can be occasions when disagreements arise regarding the best course of treatment. This is often challenging, requiring delicate communication and a clear understanding of the medical facts. However, it's essential to stand our ground when we believe a patient's needs are not being met. We must become empowered to advocate for our patients to ensure that their voice is heard when they aren't able to speak for themselves.

One memorable case involved a patient, Ms. Garcia, who had been experiencing persistent chest pain. The hospital physician, after an initial examination, attributed it to musculoskeletal pain and recommended over-the-counter analgesics. However, based on Ms. Garcia's presentation and my experience, I felt the pain warranted a more thorough cardiac investigation. I voiced my concerns to the attending physician, providing a detailed account of Ms. Garcia's symptoms and vital signs, stressing the necessity of a more comprehensive workup, even if it meant pushing for additional diagnostics. My persistence led to a more thorough evaluation, ultimately revealing a significant cardiac issue. Had I not advocated for Ms. Garcia, her condition could have deteriorated significantly.

Advocating for patients often involves navigating complex healthcare systems and insurance procedures. We're often the first point of contact for patients in crisis, and our understanding of the healthcare landscape can significantly impact their outcome. This means working closely with hospital personnel, insurance companies, and social services, always with the goal of streamlining the process to ensure patients receive the best care.

This often involves working with the hospital staff to ensure a smooth transition of care. This includes relaying accurate and complete patient information, including their medical history, current condition, medication list, and any allergies. This seamless handover of information is vital to prevent any delays or errors in treatment. A clear and concise handover report is essential. It's not just about providing details; it's about ensuring the team receiving the patient is well-prepared to continue their care without any interruption. It is an intricate dance between effective communication and a deep understanding of the importance of the patient's needs.

On several occasions, I've had to act as a bridge between patients who struggle to communicate their needs and the healthcare system designed to support them. Many patients lack the necessary knowledge or resources to navigate the complex world of healthcare. This might involve helping patients understand their medical bills, finding financial assistance programs, or connecting them with social workers or case managers. We're not just paramedics; we're often the link connecting vulnerable individuals to the resources they need. We are the advocates, the bridge between their suffering and the hope of recovery. It is often this small gesture of empathy and guidance that makes the biggest impact.

Effective patient advocacy requires a multifaceted approach. It demands a deep understanding of medical practices, legal rights, and the social determinants of health. It requires strong communication skills, the ability to navigate complex systems, and the confidence to stand up for what is right, even when facing resistance. Yet, it's also rooted in empathy and compassion, in understanding the vulnerability and anxieties of those we serve. It's about building trust, creating space for open communication and ensuring that patients feel empowered to participate in their own healthcare decisions. It's a testament to our commitment to putting the patient first, always.

In conclusion, advocating for patients is not just a part of the job; it is the heart of our work. It's about going beyond the immediate medical response to become a champion for our patients, ensuring they receive the quality of care they deserve, regardless of their circumstances. It's a responsibility we embrace, not as a burden, but as a privilege. It is the fulfillment of our oath – to serve, to protect, and most importantly, to advocate for those in our care. It's a commitment to the humanity at the core of paramedicine, a commitment that keeps us returning to the job, time and time again, despite its challenges. It's the essence of what makes this challenging, rewarding, and deeply meaningful profession so fulfilling.

7

Legal and Ethical Considerations in Paramedicine

The previous section highlighted the crucial role of patient advocacy in paramedicine, emphasizing the moral and ethical obligations we have to ensure our patients receive the best possible care. This advocacy, however, must always operate within clearly defined legal boundaries. Understanding and respecting these boundaries is paramount not only for our patients' safety but also for our own professional protection. This section delves into the intricacies of our scope of practice, exploring the legal framework that governs our actions and the potential consequences of exceeding its limitations.

Our scope of practice isn't a static entity; it's a dynamic interplay between state and local regulations, institutional policies, and our individual levels of certification and training. It's not simply a list of procedures we can perform; it's a complex web of legal permissions and restrictions that dictate what we are authorized to do, where we can do it, and under what circumstances. This complexity makes it crucial for every paramedic to regularly review and update their understanding of these regulations. Neglecting this can have serious legal and professional repercussions.

One key aspect of our scope of practice is the concept of "standard of care." This is the level of skill and care that a reasonably prudent paramedic would provide in a similar situation. It's not about perfection; it's about acting in a manner consistent with established best practices and accepted medical protocols. Deviation from this standard, without justifiable reason, can lead to allegations of negligence or malpractice. This standard is constantly evolving, reflecting advancements in medical technology and knowledge. Staying abreast of these changes through continuing education and professional development is crucial to maintaining compliance and delivering optimal patient care.

For example, a failure to utilize a newly available defibrillation device or the application of a recently developed airway management technique can be viewed as a deviation from the standard of care, depending on circumstances and availability. A paramedic who makes the decision not to use a life-saving technique available to them could face serious legal consequences if the patient's outcome could have been improved. The same would apply in other situations, where updated best practices are not followed. This highlights the responsibility we have not just to provide medical treatment, but also to continually update our practices and knowledge.

The legal parameters of our actions are particularly critical when considering the administration of medications. Each medication we carry has specific protocols and indications for use. Administering a medication outside these guidelines, even with seemingly good intentions, can expose us to liability. This underscores the importance of meticulous documentation, accurately recording the patient's condition, the medication administered, the dosage, the route of administration, and the observed response. Thorough documentation isn't simply a bureaucratic requirement; it's a crucial element in defending our actions if legal challenges arise.

A personal anecdote underscores this point. Early in my career, I responded to a call involving a patient experiencing severe respiratory distress. I felt strongly that a particular medication would help and therefore, administered it. However, I did not properly document the rationale and process of my decision. I later faced intense scrutiny when an adverse event occurred, even though my actions were ultimately justified. The lack of meticulous documentation almost compromised my defense, even though my decision to administer the medication was later deemed appropriate by a panel of experts. This event drilled into my memory the life-long lesson on the significance of detailed and comprehensive documentation. It's a cornerstone of legal protection, regardless of the immediate justification of our actions.

Another significant area within our scope of practice is the ability to perform invasive procedures. Depending on certification and state regulations, paramedics might be authorized to perform endotracheal intubation, intraosseous access, and cardioversion. However, the ability to perform such procedures comes with corresponding responsibilities and legal limitations. Each procedure has specific guidelines and indications, and performing it improperly or in an inappropriate context can have serious consequences. This again emphasizes the need for ongoing training, meticulous adherence to protocols, and precise documentation.

Beyond the specific procedures we're permitted to perform, our scope of practice also dictates the authority we have in making clinical decisions. We have the right, and often the responsibility, to assess a patient's condition, make a diagnosis, and decide on a plan of treatment. However, this authority is bounded by our training, experience, and the resources available to us. It is crucial for us to always act with humility and awareness of our limitations. If we are uncertain about a patient's condition or the appropriate course of action, it is paramount to seek consultation from a medical director or a more senior colleague.

There have been occasions when I hesitated about the best course of action with a patient, and instead of acting without full confidence, I chose to consult a superior. The outcome was usually positive and often far exceeded my initial expectations. The patient received the best possible care, which avoided potential risks.

Furthermore, our scope of practice extends beyond clinical skills and involves legal responsibilities. We must understand and comply with laws related to patient confidentiality, informed consent, and the reporting of certain events such as suspected child abuse or domestic violence. Violating these laws can have significant legal repercussions, both professionally and personally. It's imperative to be fully aware of not just our medical responsibilities, but our ethical and legal obligations regarding patient rights and community safety.

For instance, the Health Insurance Portability and Accountability Act (HIPAA) sets stringent standards regarding patient privacy. Disclosing protected health information without authorization, even with seemingly harmless intentions, can have serious consequences. A simple seemingly minor breach of this legislation can result in fines, suspensions, or even criminal charges.

Finally, maintaining a current understanding of our scope of practice requires ongoing professional development. The medical field is constantly evolving, and with it, our scope of practice may also shift. Through participation in continuing education courses, attending conferences, and engaging in self-directed learning, we can stay abreast of these changes and ensure that our actions remain within legal and ethical boundaries. The paramedic profession demands a commitment to continuous learning; it's not enough to simply meet the minimum requirements; we have a responsibility to strive for excellence in all aspects of our work.

In summary, understanding and adhering to the legal scope of practice is fundamental to the safe and effective delivery of pre-hospital care. It requires not only a thorough understanding of regulations and protocols but also a commitment to ongoing professional development and meticulous documentation. Operating within these defined boundaries protects both our patients and ourselves, ensuring that we provide high-quality care while upholding the integrity of our profession. This is more than just a set of rules; it's a commitment to responsible and ethical practice, underpinning everything we do as paramedics. By staying informed and consistently striving to improve our knowledge and skills, we remain committed to both our patients' well-being and the ethical practice of our demanding and critical profession.

Informed consent is the cornerstone of ethical and legal paramedic practice. It represents the patient's voluntary agreement to receive medical treatment, based on a thorough understanding of the procedure, its potential benefits, risks, and alternatives. This understanding is crucial; a patient's consent obtained without full disclosure is invalid, exposing us to potential legal ramifications. The legal implications are significant; providing treatment without informed consent can constitute battery, a serious legal offense. The principle of autonomy, a core tenet of medical ethics, underlines the patient's right to make decisions about their own body and health. Our role as paramedics is not to impose treatment, but to facilitate informed choices.

The process of obtaining informed consent isn't a simple checklist; it's a dynamic interaction requiring clear communication, empathy, and a keen awareness of the patient's mental capacity and circumstances. It's essential to assess the patient's ability to understand the information presented, their level of cognitive function, and any language barriers. For instance, a patient suffering from a severe head injury may lack the cognitive capacity to provide informed consent. In such cases, alternative means of consent, such as implied consent or consent from a legal guardian, may be necessary. Implied consent comes into play when a patient's condition prevents explicit consent but immediate treatment is necessary to prevent death or serious harm. This is a high-stakes scenario, and careful judgment is essential.

My own experience highlights the nuances of this process. During a night shift, we responded to a call involving a young man experiencing a severe seizure. He was unresponsive and his breathing was labored. Given the urgency, I initiated advanced life support, invoking implied consent. The situation clearly necessitated immediate intervention; delaying treatment to wait for explicit consent would have risked permanent brain damage, or even death. However, post-incident review was critical, as we were required to document that we had considered implied consent appropriately. The detailed documentation, outlining the patient's condition and the urgency of the situation, was vital in justifying our actions. This experience reinforced the critical relationship between timely intervention and a thorough record, providing a robust defense in potentially challenging circumstances.

Obtaining consent from a patient with cognitive impairments or a language barrier requires additional care and attention. We must adapt our communication strategies to ensure understanding. This could involve using visual aids, translating services, or seeking the assistance of family members or interpreters. In situations where a patient is incapacitated or mentally incapable, the process often involves securing consent from a designated legal guardian or surrogate decision-maker, adhering strictly to the legal requirements dictated by the patient's location and the jurisdiction in which we are practicing. These situations often demand patience and clarity in communicating with the legal guardians.

The level of information provided should be tailored to the patient's capacity to understand, considering their medical literacy and cognitive abilities. Overwhelming the patient with complex medical jargon can hinder the informed consent process. The information shared should be presented in plain language, and the patient should be given the opportunity to ask questions and express their concerns. We need to explain the procedure and treatment plan in a clear, straightforward manner, avoiding technical jargon. This is paramount to ensure true comprehension and informed consent.

Furthermore, the information disclosed must encompass not just the potential benefits of the treatment but also the associated risks, including the possibility of adverse effects or complications. Omitting information about potential risks, however unlikely, invalidates the consent. A crucial element of this discussion is also presenting viable alternatives, if they exist. For example, when considering administering a particular medication, we are obligated to discuss potential alternatives or alternative treatment pathways if available. Transparency and honesty are paramount. Honest discussion about risk mitigation also plays a key role. This includes providing information regarding how we plan to minimize potential risks and manage potential complications.

Documenting the informed consent process is equally crucial. Detailed records of the conversation, the information provided, the patient's questions and concerns, and the ultimate decision regarding treatment are vital for legal protection and for clear continuity of care. The documentation should indicate the patient's competence to make decisions and understanding of the procedure and associated risks. The lack of sufficient and appropriate documentation can easily lead to serious problems. My own experience as a paramedic emphasizes this point. I have witnessed cases where well-intentioned treatment was jeopardized by inadequate documentation, leading to questioning of procedures and subsequent legal complications for colleagues.

Specific circumstances, such as situations involving minors or patients under the influence of drugs or alcohol, demand even greater care and attention to detail. Obtaining consent for a minor requires the involvement of a parent or legal guardian. This situation requires careful assessment of the parent or guardian's legal authority and their under-standing of the proposed treatment plan. In the case of a patient under the influence of drugs or alcohol, the ability to provide informed con-sent may be impaired. In this situation, we need to carefully assess their mental capacity, their understanding of the treatment, and the need for immediate intervention. This often requires a delicate balance between providing life-saving care and respecting the individual's rights.

The legal landscape surrounding informed consent can vary from ju-risdiction to jurisdiction. It's crucial to be familiar with the specific state and local laws and regulations governing the provision of pre-hospital care. Regular professional development and staying informed about le-gal and ethical updates are essential. This highlights the continuing ed-ucational needs within the profession to remain abreast of changes in regulations and best practices. This continuous learning is more than just a professional obligation; it's a commitment to the ethical and safe delivery of emergency medical services. It safeguards both the patient and the paramedic.

Ultimately, obtaining informed consent is more than just a legal re-quirement; it's an ethical obligation. It reflects our respect for patient autonomy, our commitment to providing safe and effective care, and our responsibility to uphold the highest standards of professional prac-tice. It's a continuous process demanding clear communication, empa-thy, and a deep understanding of both the legal and ethical principles governing pre-hospital care. The process is not merely a box to be ticked; it's a foundation on which our patient-centered approach is built, en-hancing both safety and trust.

The ethical duty to protect patient confidentiality extends far be-yond a simple sense of professional decorum; it forms the bedrock of trust between patient and provider, a trust essential for effective health-care. This responsibility is codified in law, most notably through the

Health Insurance Portability and Accountability Act (HIPAA) in the United States, which establishes stringent regulations for the protection of Protected Health Information (PHI). Understanding and adhering to these regulations isn't simply a matter of avoiding legal repercussions; it's a fundamental aspect of upholding the patient's right to privacy and dignity.

HIPAA's reach encompasses a wide array of patient information, including anything that can be used to identify an individual and relate to their past, present, or future physical or mental health or condition. This includes seemingly innocuous details like a patient's name, address, date of birth, social security number, medical records, and even the fact that they are receiving treatment at a particular location. The breadth of this definition underscores the pervasive nature of PHI and the vigilance required in its protection.

The penalties for HIPAA violations can be significant, ranging from civil monetary penalties to criminal prosecution, depending on the nature and severity of the violation. These penalties are not merely theoretical threats; they represent a real and substantial risk to individual paramedics and to the organizations they work for. The financial ramifications can be crippling, and the reputational damage can be long-lasting, impacting both career prospects and public trust.

Beyond the legal repercussions, breaches of confidentiality can have profound ethical and emotional consequences for patients. The violation of their trust can undermine their willingness to be open and honest with healthcare providers, hindering the ability to provide effective care. This breach of trust can lead to feelings of vulnerability, anxiety, and even fear, potentially impacting their future willingness to seek medical attention. In sensitive cases, such as those involving mental health or substance abuse, a breach of confidentiality can have particularly devastating effects.

In my experience, even seemingly minor breaches of confidentiality can have unforeseen consequences. I recall a situation where an offhand remark about a patient's condition to a colleague in the break room – a remark intended to be innocuous and quickly forgotten – inadvertently led to the patient's identity being revealed within their close-knit community. The patient, who had a history of substance abuse, faced further social stigma and challenges as a result, a stark reminder of the potentially far-reaching implications of even casual disclosures.

Maintaining HIPAA compliance requires a multifaceted approach, encompassing robust administrative, physical, and technical safeguards. Administrative safeguards involve establishing clear policies and procedures for handling PHI, including protocols for access, use, disclosure, and disposal of patient information. These policies should be regularly reviewed and updated to reflect changes in legislation and best practices. Training is paramount; all personnel handling PHI must receive comprehensive training on HIPAA regulations and the importance of patient confidentiality. Regular refresher courses are equally essential to ensure continued understanding and adherence.

Physical safeguards address the protection of paper-based records and other physical materials containing PHI. This includes measures such as secure storage of medical records, locked file cabinets, and access controls to limit physical access to sensitive information. The handling of medical records should also be carefully controlled; only authorized individuals should have access to a patient's medical records, and these individuals should be thoroughly vetted for reliability and trustworthiness. Furthermore, the disposal of medical records must comply with established guidelines to ensure confidentiality after the records are no longer needed.

Technical safeguards are critical in the digital age, where PHI is increasingly stored and transmitted electronically. This includes the use of secure electronic health records (EHRs) systems, strong passwords, encryption protocols, and access control mechanisms to limit access to PHI based on the user's role and responsibilities. Firewalls and intrusion detection systems are essential for protecting EHR systems from unauthorized access and cyberattacks. Regular system backups and disaster recovery planning are also crucial for safeguarding patient information in case of system failures or other disruptions.

The use of electronic devices, such as tablets and smartphones, in the pre-hospital setting requires specific attention to HIPAA compliance. These devices often contain sensitive patient information, and their loss or theft could result in a major security breach. The use of such devices should be strictly controlled, and employees should be educated on the importance of secure device management and data protection. It is paramount that all devices are secured against unauthorized access and that sensitive patient information is encrypted when stored on such devices.

Furthermore, the transmission of PHI via electronic means, such as email or fax, demands rigorous security protocols. All electronic communications containing PHI should be encrypted to protect the information from interception. Employees must also be educated on the appropriate use of electronic communication for PHI, including the importance of avoiding unsecured communication channels. It's important to remember that even seemingly innocuous email headers can inadvertently disclose PHI.

The concept of "minimum necessary" is central to HIPAA compliance. It mandates that only the minimum amount of PHI necessary to accomplish a specific purpose be accessed, used, or disclosed. This principle underscores the importance of limiting access to patient information to only those individuals who have a legitimate need to know, reducing the risk of inadvertent or intentional disclosures. This requires careful consideration of the information required for each task, and avoiding unnecessary data retrieval and sharing.

The responsibility for HIPAA compliance rests not only on individual paramedics but also on the organizations that employ them. EMS agencies must establish comprehensive HIPAA compliance programs, including policies, procedures, training, and oversight mechanisms. Regular audits and risk assessments are essential for identifying and addressing potential vulnerabilities in the system. These programs must actively monitor adherence to established procedures and protocols to maintain a high level of compliance. Any identified non-compliance must be addressed promptly and effectively.

The penalties for non-compliance can extend beyond the immediate financial and legal ramifications. The erosion of public trust and the damage to the reputation of the EMS agency can have long-term consequences. It can significantly impact the organization's ability to attract and retain qualified personnel and may hinder the organization's ability to secure funding and contracts. These considerations add urgency to the need for robust and effective HIPAA compliance programs.

Effective communication is key to preventing breaches of confidentiality. Paramedics should be trained to communicate sensitive patient information only to authorized individuals using appropriate channels. They should be aware of the potential risks of discussing patient information in public places or with unauthorized individuals. The use of coded language or euphemisms should be avoided, as it can lead to misunderstandings and potential breaches. A culture of confidentiality, where employees understand the importance of protecting patient privacy, is paramount.

Ultimately, upholding patient confidentiality is more than just a legal obligation; it is a moral imperative. It reflects the commitment of paramedics to providing compassionate, ethical, and trustworthy care. By adhering to HIPAA regulations and prioritizing the protection of patient information, paramedics not only fulfill their legal and ethical duties but also strengthen the essential bonds of trust that underpin the patient-provider relationship. This trust, hard-earned and easily broken, is the lifeblood of effective and ethical paramedicine. It's not merely a box to tick; it's a foundational pillar of the profession.

Accurate and complete documentation is not merely a matter of good practice; it's a legal imperative. The paramedic's record serves as the primary source of information regarding a patient's condition, the care provided, and the overall events of the call.

This record becomes crucial evidence in potential legal disputes, insurance claims, and even criminal investigations. Inaccurate, incomplete, or missing documentation can have significant legal repercussions, potentially leading to accusations of negligence, malpractice, or even criminal charges. It's a stark reality that a poorly maintained record can unravel even the most meticulously executed patient care.

The legal standards surrounding paramedic documentation vary by jurisdiction, but the core principle remains consistent: the record must accurately reflect the events of the call and the care administered. This means meticulously recording the patient's chief complaint, vital signs, assessment findings, interventions performed, and the patient's response to treatment. Omitting details, making inaccurate entries, or falsifying information are serious offenses that can have lasting consequences.

One common pitfall is the temptation to rely on memory. The adrenaline-fueled environment of an emergency call can make it difficult to remember every detail, especially with a high volume of calls during peak hours or in high-stress situations. However, relying on memory is a dangerous gamble. Details that may seem trivial at the time can become crucial pieces of evidence later on. This is why diligent note-taking, even in the midst of chaos, is paramount. I vividly remember a call involving a head injury; the initial assessment seemed routine, but a detail about the patient's diminished responsiveness later became crucial when a legal challenge questioned the adequacy of care. Had I been less diligent in documenting that specific observation, I could have faced serious repercussions.

Moreover, the documentation must be timely. Delayed documentation can raise serious questions about its accuracy and reliability, making it less credible in legal proceedings. The immediacy of recording events ensures that the details are fresh in the mind, and the risk of errors or omissions is minimized. Many EMS agencies have specific protocols for documenting patient information within a short timeframe after the call ends, often using electronic systems that automatically timestamp the entries, providing a verifiable audit trail.

Beyond accuracy and timeliness, the documentation must be legible. Illegible handwriting, ambiguous abbreviations, or poorly organized notes can be detrimental in a legal context. A judge or jury will likely not appreciate having to decipher cryptic medical jargon under pressure. Clarity and precision in record-keeping are paramount. EMS agencies are increasingly implementing electronic documentation systems to address the challenges posed by illegible handwriting. These systems often have pre-defined options and templates that help to ensure consistency and minimize ambiguity.

The use of standardized terminology and abbreviations is equally important. Using clear, consistent language reduces the risk of misinterpretations and ensures that the record is readily understandable to other healthcare professionals. However, non-standard abbreviations or unique jargon should be avoided unless they are clearly defined within the system. In my years of service, I've encountered instances where idiosyncratic abbreviations led to misunderstandings and created unnecessary confusion for subsequent medical personnel involved in patient care.

Another critical aspect of paramedic documentation is the appropriate use of quotation marks. When documenting a patient's statements, direct quotes should be carefully used and accurately transcribed. This prevents misinterpretation of the patient's words and maintains the integrity of the record. In situations involving potential legal disputes or accusations of patient misconduct, the patient's own words can be instrumental in clarifying the events. The importance of this detail is often underscored in legal proceedings.

Furthermore, the documentation must reflect the overall picture of the patient encounter, including any challenges faced during the call, such as difficult access to the patient's location, uncooperative bystanders, or a lack of essential equipment. These contextual factors can influence the care provided and need to be included in the documentation to provide a complete picture of the situation. Such challenges can sometimes be overlooked, but including them shows a holistic understanding of the call and the limitations faced. The patient's response to treatment, along with any complications or adverse reactions, must also be meticulously documented. These details can be significant in assessing the effectiveness of the provided care.

The legal implications of inadequate documentation extend beyond individual liability to encompass the entire EMS agency. Failure to maintain accurate and complete records can expose the agency to legal actions, reputational damage, and potential sanctions. EMS agencies are expected to have robust quality assurance and control mechanisms to ensure that their paramedics are properly trained in documentation procedures and adhere to established standards. Regular audits and reviews of documentation are essential to identify and address any deficiencies in practice.

In conclusion, proper documentation and record-keeping in paramedicine is not a mere administrative task; it's a crucial legal and ethical responsibility. It demands meticulous attention to detail, accuracy, timeliness, and clarity. The consequences of inadequate documentation can range from professional sanctions to legal repercussions, affecting not only the individual paramedic but also the EMS agency. A well-maintained record, therefore, is not just a testament to good practice but an essential safeguard against potential legal challenges and a vital component of providing high-quality and legally defensible patient care. It's a responsibility we wear alongside our stethoscopes and equipment; a responsibility we embrace for the safe and well-being of our patients and ourselves.

Beyond accurate documentation, minimizing legal exposure in paramedicine requires a multifaceted approach encompassing adherence to established protocols, prioritizing patient safety, and proactively managing risks. This involves a deep understanding of the legal landscape and a commitment to ethical practice at every stage of patient interaction.

One critical aspect is strict adherence to established protocols and standard operating procedures (SOPs). These protocols, developed by medical experts and regulatory bodies, provide a framework for consistent and evidence-based care. Deviation from these protocols, without justifiable medical reasons meticulously documented, can significantly increase the risk of legal liability. For instance, administering a medication outside the approved parameters, without appropriate documentation of the clinical rationale and informed consent, could expose a paramedic to accusations of negligence. This extends beyond medication administration to encompass all aspects of patient care, including assessment, treatment selection, and transport decisions. Regular review and updating of these protocols are crucial in keeping pace with evolving medical knowledge and best practices. Any changes in protocols necessitate thorough training for all personnel to ensure consistent understanding and implementation.

Practicing safely is paramount to mitigating legal risk. This involves a proactive approach to risk assessment and mitigation. Before engaging in any procedure, a paramedic should thoroughly assess the potential risks and implement appropriate safeguards. This might involve utilizing personal protective equipment (PPE) appropriately, ensuring adequate scene safety, and requesting additional support when necessary. I recall an incident where a seemingly straightforward motor vehicle accident rapidly escalated due to an unexpected hazardous materials spill. Our initial risk assessment had not accounted for this possibility, and our subsequent response needed to adapt quickly. By implementing additional safety measures and requesting specialized hazmat teams, we mitigated the risk to ourselves and the patient. This incident highlighted the importance of continuously reevaluating the situation and adjusting our approach as new information becomes available.

Regular equipment checks and maintenance are also crucial components of safe practice. Malfunctioning equipment can compromise patient safety and increase the risk of legal repercussions. Ensuring that all equipment is in good working order, properly calibrated, and maintained according to manufacturer recommendations is essential. A broken defibrillator or an unreliable oxygen tank can have catastrophic consequences and lead to serious legal consequences. Detailed logs of equipment maintenance and checks should be maintained as part of the overall risk management strategy.

Effective communication with patients and their families is another essential aspect of minimizing legal exposure. Obtaining informed consent before any intervention is not simply a matter of ticking a box on a form; it's about engaging in an open and honest dialogue about the risks and benefits of various treatments. This is particularly critical in cases where the patient's capacity to make decisions is compromised. In such situations, involving family members or legal guardians in the decision-making process, while adhering to relevant legal and ethical guidelines, becomes vital. I remember a case involving an elderly patient with diminished cognitive capacity. We carefully explained the necessary treatment to both the patient and their family, taking the time to answer all questions and ensuring they understood the risks and benefits before proceeding. This careful approach ensured that we not only provided appropriate care but also minimized the potential for later legal challenges.

Beyond patient communication, effective communication with other healthcare professionals is critical. Clear and concise handover reports, including a detailed summary of the patient's condition, treatment provided, and any relevant information, are paramount when transferring care to hospital staff. Miscommunication during handover can have serious consequences and could lead to legal challenges. Using standardized reporting systems, clear terminology, and written documentation minimizes the risk of ambiguity and ensures that all essential information is accurately transmitted. In this era of electronic health records (EHRs), seamless integration and data transfer between different healthcare systems become particularly important for minimizing gaps in information and preventing inconsistencies.

Continuing professional development (CPD) is equally vital in mitigating legal risk. Paramedics must stay abreast of the latest advances in medical practice, legal regulations, and ethical guidelines. Regular participation in training courses, workshops, and conferences helps to enhance skills, knowledge, and awareness of potential legal pitfalls. Staying updated on the changes in emergency medical guidelines and legal frameworks allows paramedics to provide the best possible care and reduces the risk of liability. This commitment to ongoing learning is not simply about maintaining professional competence; it's a commitment to minimizing risks and protecting both the paramedic and the patient.

Furthermore, establishing and maintaining a strong professional relationship with legal counsel is a proactive strategy for risk management. Having access to legal advice can provide valuable guidance in navigating complex situations and minimizing the risk of legal action. Early consultation with legal experts can help to establish best practices, ensure compliance with legal requirements, and provide informed decision-making in challenging cases. This proactive approach fosters a culture of risk awareness and encourages a cautious but decisive approach to clinical practice. It's prudent to have a well-defined legal support system before encountering complex situations rather than seeking it out amidst a crisis.

Finally, understanding and actively managing stress and burnout is crucial. High-stress environments can impair judgment and decision-making abilities, increasing the risk of errors and legal issues. Implementing effective stress management techniques, such as regular exercise, mindfulness practices, and seeking professional support, is not simply a matter of self-care; it's a crucial component of minimizing legal risk. A fatigued or emotionally compromised paramedic is more likely to make mistakes, increasing the chances of accidents and potential legal challenges. Prioritizing mental well-being, therefore, is not a luxury; it's a necessity for maintaining professional competence and protecting both ourselves and our patients. This holistic approach underscores that minimizing legal exposure isn't just about technical skills and procedural adherence; it's about creating a culture of continuous learning, proactive risk management, and unwavering attention to ethical practices. It's a commitment to excellence that protects the paramedics, their patients, and their profession as a whole.

8

Working in a System: The Paramedic's Role

The seamless transfer of a patient from the pre-hospital environment to the controlled setting of a hospital emergency department is a critical juncture in their care. This handoff, often occurring under immense time pressure and with multiple medical professionals involved, demands meticulous attention to detail and a high level of inter-professional collaboration. The efficiency and clarity of this transition directly impacts patient outcomes, potentially influencing the speed of diagnosis, treatment initiation, and overall prognosis. My own experience has underscored the profound impact of a well-executed handoff, contrasting sharply with instances where communication breakdowns have led to delays and potentially compromised care.

One of the cornerstone elements of a successful hospital handoff is the pre-hospital documentation. Comprehensive and accurate documentation, started at the very first patient contact, lays the foundation for a smooth and informed transfer of care. This goes far beyond simply recording vital signs and treatment administered; it necessitates a clear and concise narrative that encapsulates the patient's presentation, the paramedic's assessment, the interventions employed, and the patient's response. Using a standardized reporting format, often dictated by local protocols and hospital systems, allows for a uniform and readily understandable approach, minimizing ambiguity and facilitating quick comprehension by receiving physicians and nurses. Details such as the patient's chief complaint, allergies, pertinent medical history, current medications, and any pertinent social history become invaluable pieces of the puzzle for the receiving hospital team.

Beyond the factual data, the narrative portion of the report demands careful consideration. It's not merely a chronological listing of events, but rather a story that paints a picture of the patient's condition and their journey leading up to arrival at the hospital. It should convey the paramedic's clinical reasoning, the rationale behind treatment decisions, and any particular nuances of the case. For example, a subtle change in the patient's mental status or a seemingly innocuous detail from the scene might provide a critical clue for the hospital team's diagnostic efforts. I remember a case where a seemingly simple fall resulted in a head injury that initially presented with only subtle symptoms, yet the subtle changes in the patient's behavior documented pre-hospital were crucial in expediting the hospital team's assessment and initiating prompt neuroimaging.

Technological advancements play a significant role in streamlining this information exchange. Electronic health records (EHRs) and pre-hospital data systems have begun to improve the transfer of information, allowing for near real-time access to crucial patient data. However, even with advanced technology, human interaction remains paramount. The verbal handover, executed alongside the written report, allows for a nuanced exchange of information that transcends mere data transfer. This verbal exchange is an opportunity to convey the 'gestalt' of the patient's condition – the subtle cues, the unspoken concerns, and the overall impression formed by the paramedic during their assessment and interaction with the patient.

The verbal handover, ideally performed face-to-face or via a secure video conferencing system, should adhere to structured protocols to ensure nothing vital is overlooked. Using a standardized approach, such as the SBAR (Situation, Background, Assessment, Recommendation) method, aids in clarity and efficiency. The situation provides a concise overview of the current emergency; the background contextualizes the patient's history and leading up to the emergency; the assessment details the paramedic's findings; and the recommendation offers guidance on immediate interventions required by the hospital team. This structured format minimizes ambiguity and ensures all crucial information is conveyed. It is equally critical that the receiving physician or nurse actively participate in the handover, not just passively listening. Questions and clarifications should be openly encouraged to ensure a shared understanding.

Another critical element often overlooked is the importance of nonverbal communication during the handoff. The paramedic's demeanor, tone of voice, and body language can subtly but significantly influence how the receiving team perceives the urgency and complexity of the case. A confident, clear, and concise delivery fosters trust and confidence, whereas a hesitant or uncertain presentation could hinder a timely and effective response. I've observed firsthand how a paramedic's subtle cues, beyond the verbal report, can significantly alter the hospital team's approach – a heightened sense of concern reflected in their tone can immediately trigger a more rapid response.

Moreover, the hospital protocols themselves are vital components of efficient patient transfer. Hospitals generally have well-defined protocols that dictate the process of receiving patients from EMS. These protocols define procedures for triaging, assessment, and immediate treatment, ensuring a consistent and systematic approach. Understanding and adhering to these protocols is paramount for paramedics, as it facilitates seamless integration into the hospital workflow.

Familiarity with these protocols minimizes delays and ensures the patient receives timely and appropriate care. Regular training and collaborative exercises between EMS and hospital staff should be implemented to ensure everyone is knowledgeable about the process and procedures.

Hospital protocols can also outline specific communication methods, including designated personnel for receiving handoffs and standardized reporting forms. Adhering to these established communication channels avoids confusion and ensures that crucial information reaches the appropriate personnel efficiently. Lack of familiarity with hospital protocols can create significant delays, potentially compromising patient care. A joint effort between hospital staff and paramedic services to regularly revise and refine these protocols, incorporating lessons learned from past experiences, can further refine the efficiency and effectiveness of this crucial step in the continuum of care.

The success of a hospital handoff hinges not only on efficient procedures and technological tools but also on the cultivation of a strong collaborative relationship between paramedics and hospital staff. Regular joint training exercises, inter-agency meetings, and ongoing communication channels all serve to build trust and facilitate a seamless flow of information. These interactions, extending beyond formal handoffs, foster a shared understanding of expectations, challenges, and priorities, promoting a unified approach to patient care. Furthermore, establishing open lines of communication allows for immediate feedback and problem-solving, continually improving the efficiency and quality of the patient transfer process. Regular debriefing sessions following complex cases can highlight areas of improvement and strengthen the working relationship between EMS and hospital staff, leading to a more cohesive system of care.

Beyond the immediate transfer, the post-handoff follow-up plays a crucial role in patient care and the overall efficiency of the system. This might involve periodic updates from the hospital team, providing the paramedic with information on the patient's progress, ongoing treatment, and any unexpected developments. This form of feedback not only provides closure for the paramedic but also helps identify areas for improvement in the pre-hospital care delivered. This closed-loop communication highlights the ongoing collaborative nature of patient care and supports continuous improvement in the entire healthcare system.

In conclusion, efficient patient transfer between paramedics and hospital staff demands a meticulous approach, encompassing clear and concise communication, adherence to established protocols, a strategic use of technology, and a strong inter-professional relationship. The efficiency of this transition directly impacts patient outcomes, underscoring the importance of consistent training, collaborative efforts, and an unwavering focus on seamless communication. It's a complex interplay of human interaction, established procedures, and technological advancements that ultimately determines the effectiveness of the entire healthcare continuum, impacting the health and well-being of those we serve. The ultimate goal isn't simply the physical transfer of a patient; it's the seamless continuation of high-quality, coordinated care, ensuring the best possible outcome for those in our care. This requires a continuous commitment to improvement, reflection, and ongoing collaboration among all stakeholders involved.

Effective interprofessional collaboration is not merely a desirable trait in emergency medical services; it's the bedrock upon which the entire system rests. Our success, and more importantly, the well-being of our patients, hinges on our ability to seamlessly integrate with other healthcare providers. This extends beyond the simple handoff in the emergency room; it encompasses ongoing communication and collaboration throughout the entire patient journey. I've seen firsthand the difference between a well-oiled machine of coordinated care and a fragmented system where communication breakdowns lead to delays and potentially disastrous outcomes.

One crucial area of collaboration involves working with emergency department physicians. These are the individuals who will ultimately make the critical diagnostic and treatment decisions after receiving the patient from our care. Building rapport with the ED physicians is essential. This isn't just about exchanging information efficiently; it's about establishing trust and mutual respect. This trust is forged over time through consistent professionalism, accurate reporting, and a willingness to engage in open dialogue. I recall one instance where a seasoned ED physician, after a particularly complex cardiac arrest, expressed his appreciation for my detailed pre-hospital report, highlighting how it facilitated quicker diagnosis and treatment. That shared moment of understanding, built on a foundation of effective collaboration, was profoundly satisfying. It highlighted the impact we have beyond the immediate scene; our actions have cascading effects that ripple throughout the healthcare continuum.

Beyond the initial handoff, maintaining communication with the ED team is crucial, especially in complex cases. Promptly addressing their questions, offering updates on evolving conditions, and being available for consultation demonstrates our commitment to the patient's well-being even after we've left the scene. This ongoing collaboration fosters a sense of shared responsibility, ensuring that the patient receives a unified and coordinated approach to care. One particular experience involves a patient with a severe head injury who initially presented with subtle signs. My detailed report and subsequent phone call with the neurosurgeon, offering updates on the patient's changing condition, facilitated the immediate commencement of life-saving neurosurgical intervention. This illustrates the critical role of ongoing collaboration beyond the initial ED handoff.

Our relationship extends beyond physicians. Nurses represent a significant link in the chain of care, often the first point of contact for the patient upon arrival at the hospital. Effective communication with the nursing staff is crucial for ensuring a smooth transition and facilitating the prompt initiation of treatment. This includes sharing not just the vital signs and treatment history but also offering insight into the patient's demeanor, responses, and any unique observations made in the pre-hospital setting. A simple comment about the patient's anxiety level or their response to pain medication can provide invaluable context for the nursing team, aiding in their assessment and care.

Furthermore, collaborating with other emergency medical services personnel is paramount. This includes dispatchers, other paramedics and EMTs, and even members of other agencies such as fire departments and police officers who might be involved in emergency response. Effective communication within our own EMS system is critical. Sharing information, coordinating resources, and maintaining a clear communication chain ensures a coordinated response to emergency situations. This often involves seamless communication with dispatchers, relaying crucial information about patient status and scene conditions. It also extends to collaborating with other paramedics or EMTs on scene, working as a cohesive team to manage complex cases effectively and safely.

Collaboration extends beyond the immediate response. Regular training exercises and inter-agency meetings provide invaluable opportunities to refine our skills and enhance our coordination. Simulations that mimic real-world scenarios allow us to practice our communication, teamwork, and overall response efficiency. These exercises are not simply about technical skills; they're about refining communication protocols and developing a shared understanding of roles and responsibilities. I've witnessed firsthand how these joint training sessions improved our response time, reduced errors, and strengthened the trust and camaraderie within our team. The shared understanding cultivated through these experiences translates to a more efficient and effective response during actual emergencies.

This inter-professional collaboration also plays a critical role in improving patient outcomes. Studies have shown that effective teamwork, clear communication, and coordinated care contribute to reduced mortality rates, shorter hospital stays, and improved patient satisfaction. These are not just abstract metrics; they represent real improvements in the lives of the people we serve. The emotional satisfaction of knowing that our coordinated efforts contribute to better patient outcomes is a powerful motivator. It underscores the value of investing in our collaborative skills and enhancing our ability to work seamlessly with others.

Beyond the clinical aspects, fostering strong interpersonal relationships with other healthcare professionals is essential. This involves building rapport, demonstrating respect, and acknowledging the expertise and contributions of everyone involved in the patient's care. It's about creating a culture of mutual respect and trust, where we recognize that we are all working towards a common goal: providing the best possible care for the patient. Simple acts of kindness, open communication, and a willingness to collaborate fosters a sense of camaraderie and teamwork, leading to more efficient and effective care delivery.

Technological advancements have also played a significant role in enhancing interprofessional collaboration. Electronic health records (EHRs), mobile data terminals, and telemedicine systems allow for seamless sharing of information, irrespective of location. These technologies facilitate timely access to crucial patient data, reducing the risk of miscommunication and delays in treatment. However, technology is merely a tool; it cannot replace the importance of direct human interaction. The personal touch, the ability to engage in open communication, and the development of strong interpersonal relationships remain essential for effective collaboration. Technology should augment, not replace, the human element of care.

Finally, reflective practice is crucial for improving interprofessional collaboration. Regular debriefing sessions following complex cases provide valuable opportunities to identify areas for improvement in communication, teamwork, and coordination. Honest self-reflection, alongside constructive feedback from colleagues, is essential for continuous learning and growth. This process allows us to learn from both our successes and failures, continuously refining our ability to work effectively within a multidisciplinary healthcare team. By critically analyzing our actions, we not only enhance our own skills, but we also contribute to a better and more coordinated healthcare system. This continuous cycle of reflection and improvement is paramount for the effective delivery of care within the complex environment of the modern healthcare system. Interprofessional collaboration is not just a skill; it is a philosophy, a commitment to working together to provide the best possible care for every patient.

The traditional image of a paramedic – lights flashing, siren wailing, racing to an emergency scene – is only part of the story. The scope of our profession is expanding rapidly, and a significant part of this evolution is community paramedicine. This isn't just about responding to 911 calls; it's about proactively engaging with our communities to improve overall health and well-being, bridging the gap between acute care and preventative medicine. It's a shift in paradigm, requiring a different mindset, a broader skill set, and a deeper understanding of the social determinants of health.

My own introduction to this evolving role came unexpectedly. During a routine call for a patient with chronic obstructive pulmonary disease (COPD), I noticed a pattern: repeated hospitalizations, often triggered by preventable factors like missed medications or inadequate home oxygen. This patient wasn't receiving the ongoing support they needed to manage their condition effectively. This sparked a conversation, and with the patient's consent, I connected them with resources

such as home healthcare nurses, respiratory therapists, and social workers. The results were striking. Hospital readmissions decreased significantly, and the patient reported a greater sense of control over their
health. This singular experience profoundly impacted my perspective
on the potential of community paramedicine.

Community paramedicine programs vary widely across the country,
but their core purpose remains consistent: enhancing healthcare access,
improving patient outcomes, and reducing healthcare costs. This is ac-
complished through a diverse range of activities, extending far beyond
emergency response. We might find ourselves conducting home health
assessments, providing medication management support, performing
routine wound care, or even conducting health screenings in underserved communities. One program I'm familiar with utilizes paramedics
to conduct post-discharge follow-ups for patients at high risk of read-
mission. This proactive approach allows us to identify potential complications early and intervene before they escalate into a crisis, saving both
the patient and the healthcare system significant resources.

The shift to this broader role requires a change in mindset. We move
from reactive, acute care to proactive, preventative medicine. This requires a deep understanding of chronic disease management, patient education, and resource navigation. It also necessitates a strong emphasis
on building rapport with patients and their families.

Trust is paramount, as we move from being short-term responders to
long-term partners in their healthcare journey. One of the most rewarding aspects of community paramedicine is the opportunity to build
meaningful, lasting relationships with patients, empowering them to
take control of their own health. This long-term relationship fosters
a different kind of interaction than the high-stress, time-constrained
emergency responses we are typically used to.

The skills needed in community paramedicine often extend beyond the traditional paramedic skillset. Strong communication and interpersonal skills are essential for building rapport and effectively educating patients. Cultural competency is crucial to navigate the diverse populations we serve, ensuring equitable access to care. A good community paramedic requires adeptness in resource coordination, connecting patients with social services, home healthcare agencies, and other relevant support systems. This ability often involves navigating complex bureaucratic systems to ensure patients receive the support they need. It also includes the ability to recognize social determinants of health, such as poverty, housing insecurity, or lack of access to transportation, which play a significant role in patients' health outcomes. Addressing these issues is often outside the scope of traditional emergency medicine but is critical to long-term patient well-being.

Technological advancements play an increasingly significant role in the effectiveness of community paramedicine programs. Mobile health (mHealth) technologies such as remote patient monitoring devices can enable paramedics to track vital signs, medication adherence, and other health parameters remotely. This allows for early identification of potential problems, preventing hospital readmissions and enhancing the overall quality of care. Telemedicine, too, has transformative potential. We can conduct virtual consultations with patients, offering guidance, education, and monitoring without requiring an in-person visit, particularly beneficial for patients with mobility issues or those living in remote areas. The efficient and secure transmission of patient data via electronic health records is crucial for seamless communication with other members of the healthcare team. This technological integration enhances efficiency and ensures a holistic approach to patient care.

Integrating community paramedics within the broader healthcare system presents unique challenges. Establishing clear protocols and pathways for referrals, billing, and documentation is crucial for the sustainability and success of such programs. Collaboration with other healthcare professionals, including physicians, nurses, social workers, and home health agencies, is paramount. It's vital to forge strong working relationships, establishing clear communication channels and shared understanding of roles and responsibilities. One common concern involves reimbursement models. Securing adequate reimbursement for the expanded services provided by community paramedics is vital. This often requires innovative approaches to billing and demonstrating the cost-effectiveness of preventative care initiatives. Addressing these administrative and logistical issues is vital to the widespread adoption and success of community paramedicine programs.

The impact of community paramedicine extends beyond individual patients. It has the potential to significantly improve population health, reduce healthcare costs, and enhance the overall efficiency of the healthcare system. Studies have shown that proactive interventions can reduce hospital readmissions, emergency department visits, and overall healthcare utilization. By addressing the social determinants of health and providing preventive care, we can create healthier communities. This in turn reduces the strain on emergency services, allowing us to focus our resources more effectively on acute emergencies. The long-term benefits of community paramedicine extend beyond the immediate patient, contributing to a healthier, more resilient community as a whole. From a broader perspective, community paramedicine represents a more cost-effective and sustainable approach to healthcare delivery. By preventing crises before they happen, we're investing in a healthier future for our communities.

Despite the significant potential, challenges remain. One key hurdle is the need for specialized training and education for paramedics who transition into these expanded roles. This includes advanced skills in chronic disease management, patient education, and social determinants of health. Further, the establishment of clear clinical pathways and guidelines is crucial to ensuring consistency and quality of care. It's vital that these programs are evidence-based, with robust data collection and evaluation systems in place to demonstrate their effectiveness and justify ongoing funding. The development of standardized protocols and guidelines is crucial for ensuring the quality and consistency of community paramedicine services across different regions.

As community paramedicine continues to evolve, we can anticipate even greater integration with other healthcare settings, such as primary care clinics and telehealth platforms. This increased interconnectedness will further enhance the efficiency and effectiveness of preventative care. We're seeing a growing recognition of the value of paramedics in coordinating care for patients with complex medical needs, bridging the gap between different levels of care. The future likely includes expanded roles, embracing further specialization within community paramedicine, potentially focusing on specific populations or conditions.

In conclusion, community paramedicine represents a significant and exciting evolution in the paramedic profession. It's a chance to move beyond the immediate emergency and engage in a more holistic approach to healthcare, improving both the lives of individual patients and the health of our communities. This paradigm shift demands a commitment to lifelong learning, adaptability, and a willingness to embrace new roles and responsibilities. The potential rewards—healthier communities, improved patient outcomes, and a more fulfilling career—are significant and well worth the ongoing effort. The journey continues, and I look forward to witnessing the continued development and impact of community paramedicine in the years to come.

The tranquil rhythm of everyday EMS calls – the steady pulse of routine medical emergencies – can be shattered in an instant. The calm predictability gives way to the chaotic crescendo of a mass casualty incident (MCI). These events, whether a natural disaster, terrorist attack, or industrial accident, demand a completely different level of preparedness, response, and resilience from paramedics. It's a stark contrast to the often solitary nature of community paramedicine, demanding a rapid shift from proactive care to reactive, life-saving interventions on a massive scale.

My first experience with an MCI was during a severe thunderstorm that ripped through our region. The sheer volume of calls was overwhelming. Trees were down, power lines snapped, and injuries ranged from minor cuts and bruises to severe trauma. The usual controlled environment of a single-patient emergency vanished, replaced by a scene of organized chaos. The initial adrenaline surge was quickly followed by a sobering realization of the scale of the disaster. We were stretched thin, resources were limited, and the need for clear, coordinated communication became paramount. This experience ingrained in me the absolute necessity of rigorous disaster preparedness.

Training for MCIs is far more than just a refresher course on basic life support. It involves rigorous simulations, often involving mock disaster scenarios, designed to replicate the high-pressure environment and logistical challenges of a real-world MCI. These exercises aren't just about honing technical skills; they're about teamwork, effective communication, and resource management under extreme stress. We practice triage – the rapid assessment and prioritization of patients based on the severity of their injuries – a critical skill in MCIs where resources are often limited. Learning to make rapid, life-or-death decisions under pressure is an integral part of this specialized training. The ability to effectively delegate tasks, coordinate with other first responders, and maintain composure in the face of overwhelming chaos is as crucial as any medical intervention.

Beyond technical skills, the psychological preparedness of paramedics is equally important. Witnessing widespread suffering and death on such a scale can have a profound impact on mental well-being. MCIs present a unique set of ethical dilemmas, forcing difficult decisions about which patients receive immediate treatment and who may have to wait. This requires a level of emotional resilience and self-awareness that's nurtured through ongoing training and debriefing sessions. The ability to manage stress, process trauma, and support one's colleagues in the aftermath of an MCI is paramount to maintaining professional well-being.

Protocols play a vital role in effective MCI response. Pre-established guidelines help to standardize procedures, ensuring consistency in the approach to triage, treatment, and patient transport. Clear communication channels are vital, utilizing a system of communication that ensures all responders are informed and coordinated. This could involve the use of specialized communication devices, designated command centers, and pre-arranged meeting points. Clear and efficient communication is vital to overcome the communication barriers that can arise in chaotic settings. A system of clear, concise reports, transmitted in a timely manner, enables efficient allocation of resources and ensures that all patients receive appropriate treatment.

The logistical challenges of MCIs are immense. The sheer number of patients needing care often overwhelms existing resources. This necessitates the development of scalable response plans, ensuring the ability to adapt to varying needs. This may involve the establishment of temporary treatment areas (TTAs), the mobilization of additional personnel and equipment, and the coordination of transportation to hospitals or other healthcare facilities. The efficient management of supplies, including medications, equipment, and even basic necessities like water and food, is crucial in the often extended duration of an MCI response.

One often overlooked aspect of MCI response is the need for post-incident support. The emotional toll on paramedics can be significant, requiring access to mental health services and peer support groups. This is crucial to help process trauma, manage stress, and prevent burnout. Regular debriefing sessions, both formal and informal, provide a crucial platform for processing experiences and fostering a sense of collective support. Addressing the emotional and psychological well-being of responders is not merely a matter of compassion; it's a vital component of ensuring their long-term effectiveness and resilience.

The integration of technology plays an increasingly vital role in MCI response. Real-time data tracking systems can provide a dynamic overview of the situation, allowing for more informed decision-making. Mobile communication devices ensure seamless communication among responders, even in areas with limited connectivity. Digital mapping and GPS tracking systems improve the efficiency of resource allocation, helping to ensure that equipment and personnel are deployed effectively to reach affected areas and patients promptly. The integration of telemedicine technologies allows for remote consultation with medical specialists, crucial in cases where expertise in specialized medical fields is needed and access to such specialists may be limited.

Collaboration with other agencies is paramount in effective MCI response. Paramedics are rarely the sole responders in large-scale incidents. Effective coordination with fire departments, law enforcement, and other emergency services, as well as hospital systems, is essential. Establishing clear lines of authority and communication protocols ensures a unified and effective approach. Joint training exercises help to streamline interagency cooperation, fostering mutual understanding and improving the overall coordination of resources. Clear protocols are needed for effective interagency communications, ensuring smooth and efficient transfer of critical information.

Disaster preparedness is not a one-time event; it's an ongoing process. Regular training, drills, and updates to protocols are essential to ensure that paramedics are adequately prepared for a range of scenarios. Continuous improvement in response strategies, based on lessons learned from past events, allows the system to evolve and adapt to the ever-changing nature of potential threats and hazards. Staying current with technological advancements and best practices ensures that paramedics have access to the latest tools and techniques to improve their effectiveness.

Beyond technical expertise and protocols, the human element of MCI response is crucial. The ability to work effectively as a team, to maintain composure under pressure, and to demonstrate empathy and compassion to those in need, is just as important as the technical skills. MCIs are not merely about managing injuries; they're about managing human lives and human suffering on a massive scale. This calls for a high level of emotional intelligence, the ability to manage stress, and the capacity for self-reflection.

In conclusion, the role of paramedics in mass casualty incidents is far-reaching and demanding, requiring specialized training, rigorous protocols, advanced technology integration, and unwavering resilience. It's a demanding yet rewarding profession, where the dedication and coordinated effort of paramedics can directly impact the outcome of life-threatening situations. The lessons learned from MCIs, both successful and challenging, continually shape and inform disaster preparedness strategies, constantly evolving to meet the ever-present threat of large-scale emergencies and creating a more robust and effective emergency response system. The commitment to continuous improvement, both individually and collectively, is the cornerstone of success in this critical aspect of paramedicine. It's a testament to the dedication and selflessness of those who serve, and the constant striving to improve the response to disasters that ultimately shapes the future of our readiness.

The landscape of healthcare is in constant flux, a dynamic ecosystem shaped by technological advancements, evolving demographics, and the ever-present pressure to improve efficiency and access. This dynamism is particularly felt within emergency medical services (EMS), a sector intrinsically linked to the broader healthcare continuum. Healthcare reform, therefore, is not just a matter of policy changes in distant government offices; it's a force that directly impacts the daily lives and work of paramedics, reshaping their roles and responsibilities in profound ways.

One major area of reform centers around the integration of EMS into broader healthcare networks. Traditionally, EMS has functioned somewhat in isolation, a rapid-response system focused on acute care and transport to hospitals. However, the current trend is towards a more seamless integration, where paramedics become active participants in a coordinated system of care, providing ongoing monitoring and management of patients, both in the pre-hospital setting and increasingly in the community. This shift requires paramedics to develop new skills and competencies, moving beyond traditional emergency interventions to encompass chronic disease management, preventative care, and patient education. I recall a particular case where, through a community paramedicine program, we were able to provide regular home health checks for an elderly patient with chronic heart failure, preventing unnecessary hospital readmissions and significantly improving the patient's quality of life. This wasn't just about responding to emergencies; it was about actively managing a patient's health over the long term. This illustrates the evolving and expanding role of paramedics in the broader healthcare landscape.

This integration also necessitates a shift in the way data is collected, managed, and utilized. Real-time data tracking of patient encounters, coupled with the increasing use of electronic health records (EHRs), allows for better analysis of patient outcomes, identification of trends, and targeted improvements in service delivery. The ability of paramedics to access and update patient records electronically fosters better communication between the pre-hospital and hospital settings, ensuring continuity of care and reducing medical errors. This data-driven approach to EMS is transforming how we understand and address health needs within the community, facilitating data-informed decision-making and resource allocation. For instance, by analyzing data on the frequency and nature of calls in specific neighborhoods, we can better target resources and proactively address underlying health issues within communities. This is the kind of preventative approach that modern healthcare reform actively pushes for.

The reimbursement models for EMS services are also undergoing significant transformation. The traditional fee-for-service model, where paramedics are paid for each individual call, is gradually giving way to value-based reimbursement systems. These models incentivize preventative care and the management of chronic conditions, rewarding EMS providers for improving patient outcomes and reducing overall healthcare costs. This requires a more strategic and data-driven approach to patient care, measuring the impact of interventions and demonstrating value to healthcare payers. This shift demands a higher level of documentation and analysis by paramedics, necessitating more comprehensive record-keeping and a greater focus on patient outcomes. The change to value-based care necessitates a move away from simply responding to calls to actively managing patient health and reducing the overall strain on the healthcare system.

Technological advancements are playing an increasingly significant role in shaping the future of EMS. The integration of telemedicine technologies allows paramedics to remotely consult with medical specialists, providing timely access to expert advice and improving patient outcomes, especially in rural or underserved areas. This is a game changer for emergency care, especially for patients who may be isolated geographically or otherwise have difficulty accessing timely medical attention. Mobile diagnostic tools, such as point-of-care testing devices, allow paramedics to perform rapid testing at the scene, enabling faster diagnosis and treatment, and potentially reducing time spent in the emergency department. These advancements streamline patient care and reduce unnecessary hospital visits, improving healthcare efficiency and accessibility. The possibilities for increased telehealth use are exciting, and may even lead to the reduction of wait times at emergency rooms. Such a change would significantly improve patient care and provide considerable relief to our overburdened emergency rooms.

The role of paramedics in the future will likely be defined not just by their skills in acute care, but also by their expertise in community health and preventative medicine. The need for enhanced training programs, emphasizing chronic disease management, public health initiatives, and community engagement, will become increasingly important. This will require a multi-faceted approach to paramedic education, integrating elements of public health, social work, and geriatric care. The ongoing development of professional standards and competency frameworks for paramedics will be essential in navigating this evolving healthcare landscape. This is not just about keeping up with medical technology but about embracing the broader community-based, holistic model that defines much of modern healthcare. This expansion of the paramedics' role necessitates a comprehensive re-evaluation of our training programs and a renewed commitment to life-long learning.

However, the integration of EMS into a broader healthcare system also presents significant challenges. One major concern is the potential for increased administrative burdens, as paramedics will be required to navigate more complex billing and documentation processes. This can lead to increased workloads, potential for burnout, and a diversion of focus from the core mission of providing patient care. There's also the need for effective data security measures to protect patient privacy and maintain the confidentiality of sensitive health information. Striking a balance between increased accountability and preventing unnecessary bureaucratic burdens will be a crucial aspect of navigating future changes. One can only hope that regulatory bodies are committed to creating systems that enhance rather than hinder effective patient care.

Another challenge is the need for adequate funding to support the expanded roles and responsibilities of paramedics. The transition to value-based care models may require significant upfront investments in training, technology, and infrastructure. Securing sufficient funding and ensuring equitable access to resources for all EMS systems will be crucial to successfully implementing these reforms. One of the great frustrations of many working in EMS is a perceived lack of political will to support EMS agencies adequately. This often creates considerable stress on those providing direct patient care. We must work toward better representation and the allocation of resources commensurate with the critical role that EMS plays in the wider healthcare ecosystem.

Finally, the mental health and well-being of paramedics remain a critical concern. The demanding nature of the job, coupled with the increased responsibilities associated with healthcare reform, could contribute to higher levels of burnout and stress. It is imperative that support systems and mental health resources remain readily accessible to paramedics, ensuring their ability to cope with the emotional toll of their work. Addressing this remains a critical task in the ongoing discussions about healthcare reform, as there can be no effective healthcare system without the well-being of its caregivers. It is often the hidden cost of healthcare that is often overlooked, the human cost. Therefore, the development of robust support systems should be a key component of any meaningful healthcare reform.

In conclusion, healthcare reform presents both opportunities and challenges for emergency medical services. The integration of EMS into broader healthcare networks, coupled with technological advancements and evolving reimbursement models, has the potential to transform the way emergency medical care is delivered. However, realizing the full potential of these reforms requires addressing the challenges of increased administrative burdens, securing adequate funding, and prioritising the mental health and well-being of paramedics. The future of EMS will be shaped by our ability to adapt to these changes, embracing innovation while maintaining a focus on patient care and the well-being of our frontline responders. The path ahead requires collaboration, innovation, and a continued commitment to improving both the quality and accessibility of emergency medical services. The dedication and resilience of paramedics, coupled with a supportive and well-funded system, are essential to ensuring the continued evolution of a strong and effective EMS infrastructure capable of meeting the healthcare needs of the future.

9

Leadership and Advocacy in Paramedicine

Developing strong leadership skills is paramount for paramedics, not just for career advancement, but for the immediate safety and well-being of patients and crew members. The chaotic, high-stakes environment of pre-hospital care demands decisive action, clear communication, and unwavering teamwork. Leading by example is the cornerstone of effective paramedic leadership, and it manifests in several key ways.

First and foremost, it means consistently demonstrating the very skills and qualities you expect from your team. This isn't about perfection; nobody is perfect, especially not in this line of work. We've all made mistakes, missed subtle signs, or experienced moments of doubt. The key is acknowledging these imperfections, learning from them, and striving to do better. I remember early in my career, rushing into a scene, adrenaline pumping, only to realize I'd forgotten a crucial piece of equipment. The resulting scramble was a valuable lesson in meticulous preparation and the importance of methodical checks. Sharing that experience with my team, not to highlight my failure, but to illustrate a teachable moment, fostered a culture of shared learning and mutual respect. This transparency builds trust and encourages a culture of open communication where mistakes are seen as opportunities for growth, not grounds for punishment.

Furthermore, leading by example means consistently upholding the highest ethical standards. This includes maintaining patient confidentiality, acting with integrity in all situations, and respecting the dignity of every individual we encounter, regardless of their circumstances. One incident stands out vividly. We responded to a call involving a homeless individual who had overdosed. The scene was chaotic and emotionally charged, yet one of my colleagues treated him with such respect and compassion. They took the time to clean him up, to speak to him calmly and reassuringly, even though he was unable to respond. That simple act of human decency profoundly affected not only the patient but also the rest of the team, demonstrating the power of empathy and professionalism in the face of adversity. This quiet leadership, the kind you demonstrate through action more than words, speaks volumes and sets an invaluable example.

Effective communication is another cornerstone of leadership. In the high-pressure world of paramedicine, clear, concise, and accurate communication can mean the difference between life and death. This encompasses more than just radio reports; it's about communicating effectively with patients, families, hospital staff, and your own team members. I've seen countless scenarios where miscommunication, or a lack thereof, nearly resulted in critical errors. For instance, a misinterpretation of a physician's instructions during a complex patient transfer could have catastrophic consequences. Leading by example in this area involves actively practicing and honing your communication skills, consistently using clear and precise language, actively listening to others, and fostering a team environment where everyone feels comfortable speaking up if they have concerns. Regular team briefings, debriefings, and simulated scenarios allow for practicing communication under various pressures, identifying weaknesses, and reinforcing best practices.

Decision-making under pressure is a critical leadership skill. Paramedics frequently find themselves making life-or-death decisions in seconds, often with incomplete information. Developing a systematic approach to decision-making, based on sound medical knowledge, careful assessment, and clear prioritization, is crucial. This involves prioritizing patient safety, maintaining composure under stress, and making informed decisions based on the available data, even if those decisions are difficult. A critical incident I recall involved a multi-casualty incident. The initial chaos was overwhelming, but our team, through our established protocols and efficient communication, was able to swiftly assess the scene, prioritize the most critical injuries, and allocate resources effectively. This wasn't luck; it was the result of consistent training and the implementation of effective leadership strategies. It highlighted the importance of pre-planning and practicing our response to critical incidents.

Beyond technical skills, emotional intelligence plays a crucial role in effective paramedic leadership. Understanding and managing your own emotions, as well as those of your team members, is essential for maintaining morale, fostering teamwork, and providing high-quality patient care. The job is emotionally taxing; we witness trauma, suffering, and loss on a regular basis. Recognizing the toll this takes on oneself and others is paramount. Creating a supportive environment, actively listening to concerns, offering encouragement, and prioritizing team well-being are all integral aspects of effective leadership. Encouraging mental health awareness and facilitating access to support resources isn't just a gesture of goodwill; it's a crucial responsibility for paramedic leaders. I've seen firsthand the devastating impact of burnout and moral injury on paramedics, and the proactive fostering of a culture of support is essential.

Furthermore, effective leadership involves empowering team members. This means fostering a collaborative environment where every member feels valued and respected, where their contributions are recognized, and where they feel empowered to speak up and share their ideas. Delegation is a key skill; effective leaders don't try to do everything themselves. They recognize the strengths of their team members and assign tasks accordingly. Providing opportunities for professional development, supporting further education, and mentoring junior colleagues are also critical. Investing in the growth of your team ultimately strengthens the entire organization. A leader who nurtures and empowers his team creates a stronger, more resilient unit, capable of meeting even the most challenging demands.

Beyond the immediate team, leadership extends to advocating for the profession as a whole. This involves actively participating in professional organizations, advocating for better working conditions, improved resources, and increased recognition for the invaluable services paramedics provide. This means being a voice for the voiceless, actively engaging in policy discussions, and ensuring that the concerns of paramedics are heard and addressed. The challenges facing EMS are numerous, from funding shortages and staffing issues to the ever-increasing complexity of patient care. Paramedics need strong advocates, leaders who are not afraid to speak out and fight for the resources and support needed to provide the highest quality of care. This advocacy not only improves the working environment for paramedics, but ultimately benefits the entire community by ensuring that high-quality EMS services remain accessible.

In conclusion, leading by example in paramedicine is a multifaceted endeavor that goes far beyond the technical skills required for the job. It involves demonstrating consistent competence, upholding ethical standards, practicing clear and effective communication, making decisive choices under pressure, fostering emotional intelligence, and empowering team members. Moreover, it extends to advocacy and the fight for better working conditions and recognition for the valuable role paramedics play in society. It requires a constant commitment to self-reflection, continuous learning, and a dedication to creating a positive and supportive environment for both colleagues and patients. The rewards, however, are immense: a highly functioning team, improved patient outcomes, and a strengthened sense of professional pride and purpose. This is a leadership model that ensures not only the survival of the EMS profession but its ongoing evolution and growth within the ever-changing landscape of modern healthcare.

Mentorship transcends simple instruction; it's about fostering a deep understanding of the profession, its inherent complexities, and the profound impact it has on both the provider and the patient. It's a reciprocal relationship, where the experienced paramedic imparts knowledge and skills, while simultaneously benefiting from the fresh perspective and enthusiasm of the new recruit. I remember my own mentor, a seasoned paramedic named Frank, who instilled in me not just the technical aspects of the job but the crucial importance of compassion, empathy, and ethical conduct. He didn't just show me how to place an IV or interpret an EKG; he demonstrated, through his actions, how to navigate the ethical gray areas, handle emotionally charged situations, and maintain composure under extreme pressure. His approach wasn't about lecturing; it was about sharing experience, demonstrating empathy, and encouraging self-reflection.

The importance of this kind of mentorship extends beyond the immediate transfer of knowledge. It's about creating a supportive environment where new paramedics feel comfortable asking questions, making mistakes, and learning from their experiences. In the high-stakes world of emergency medical services, the consequences of error can be severe. Therefore, creating a culture where open dialogue and constructive criticism are encouraged is paramount. This encourages a learning environment built on trust and respect, facilitating the safe exploration of complex scenarios, allowing newer paramedics to learn from the experiences of their mentors without the fear of repercussions.

Furthermore, effective mentoring is about more than just teaching technical skills. It involves fostering critical thinking, problem-solving skills, and clinical judgment. It's about guiding new paramedics to develop their own decision-making processes, encouraging them to consider various perspectives and to justify their actions. I regularly employed scenario-based training with my mentees. We would go through hypothetical situations, dissecting the various challenges, analyzing potential responses, and discussing the rationale behind the decision-making process. This allows for a safer environment to analyze complex medical situations, promoting collaborative problem-solving without real-world patient risk.

Beyond the clinical aspects, mentorship also plays a crucial role in preparing new paramedics for the emotional and psychological demands of the job. Paramedics regularly confront trauma, suffering, and death, and it's vital that new recruits are equipped to cope with the psychological toll. This doesn't simply involve teaching coping mechanisms; it's about fostering resilience, promoting self-awareness, and providing access to mental health resources. Openly discussing the emotional impact of the job, sharing personal experiences, and destigmatizing the pursuit of mental well-being are all vital components of effective mentoring. Sharing my own experiences with burnout and the importance of self-care helped foster an atmosphere of open communication, allowing mentees to express their concerns without judgment or fear. This encourages help-seeking behaviors and reduces the stigma often associated with mental health issues within the EMS profession.

The role of a mentor extends beyond the initial training period. It's about providing ongoing support and guidance as new paramedics navigate their careers. This includes regular check-ins, offering feedback on performance, and providing opportunities for professional development. It's about being a sounding board for challenges and celebrating successes. Mentorship is not a short-term commitment; it's an ongoing investment in the future of the profession. I've maintained close relationships with many of my mentees over the years, offering advice and guidance even after their initial training. This long-term support helps foster resilience and aids in navigating the challenges inherent to the career path.

Effective training programs play a crucial role in developing competent and compassionate paramedics. These programs should not only focus on the technical skills but also the ethical considerations, communication strategies, and the psychological aspects of pre-hospital care. Hands-on simulations, real-life scenarios, and case studies, along with regular feedback and evaluation, are crucial elements of a well-rounded curriculum. I've actively participated in developing and teaching in various paramedic training programs, always aiming to create realistic and engaging training experiences that challenge trainees and test their clinical judgement.

The emphasis on communication is paramount. Paramedics must be able to communicate effectively with patients, families, other healthcare professionals, and their colleagues. Training should incorporate scenarios requiring clear and concise communication under stressful conditions. Role-playing and simulations can help practice active listening, empathy, and the conveyance of critical information, all under simulated pressure. This skill extends to conveying information to the receiving hospitals, ensuring a smooth and efficient handover of patient care. Poor communication can lead to medical errors and potentially life-threatening situations.

Furthermore, ethical considerations should form a significant part of the training curriculum. This includes discussions of patient confidentiality, informed consent, end-of-life care, and the moral dilemmas that often arise in pre-hospital settings. These scenarios are vital to preparing future paramedics for the difficult decisions they will face. Case studies are effective teaching tools for examining potential ethical pitfalls and assessing the appropriate responses. Real-life examples can highlight the potential consequences of ethical lapses.

Effective training also involves incorporating strategies to mitigate stress and burnout. Paramedics are exposed to high levels of stress and trauma, so teaching coping mechanisms, stress management techniques, and the importance of self-care are crucial. Integrating mental health awareness into the curriculum is necessary. Destigmatizing the pursuit of help for mental health challenges is equally important and needs to be ingrained within the training program.

In addition to formal training, continuing education is essential for paramedics to stay abreast of the latest advances in medical science, treatment protocols, and emergency management techniques. Regular workshops, conferences, and online courses provide opportunities for professional development. Encouraging ongoing learning and professional growth is vital in maintaining high standards of patient care.

Training also includes the development of leadership skills, starting early in their careers. This involves teaching decision-making under pressure, teamwork, delegation, and effective communication among team members. Developing leadership skills will help future paramedics to navigate complex situations with confidence and competence. Simulations involving multiple casualties or critical incidents would allow for the honing of leadership skills in a controlled setting.

In summary, effective mentoring and comprehensive training are crucial for the development of highly skilled, compassionate, and resilient paramedics. By combining hands-on experience, simulated scenarios, ethical discussions, and stress management techniques, training programs can equip future paramedics to meet the challenges of this demanding profession. The investment in strong mentorship and robust training pays dividends in terms of improved patient care and enhanced professional well-being. The legacy of a paramedic extends far beyond individual cases; it lies in the mentoring and training of the next generation, ensuring the continuity of excellence in pre-hospital care and ultimately safeguarding the health and well-being of the communities we serve. The responsibility for fostering this continuity rests on the shoulders of experienced paramedics, demanding a profound commitment to shaping the future of the profession.

The fight for improved working conditions isn't a side hustle for paramedics; it's an integral part of our commitment to providing high-quality patient care. Burnout, understaffing, and inadequate resources directly impact our ability to perform our duties effectively and safely. We're not just advocating for ourselves; we're advocating for the patients who rely on us in their most vulnerable moments. If we're overworked, underpaid, and lacking the necessary equipment, the quality of care inevitably suffers.

My own experiences have vividly illustrated this connection. I remember a particularly grueling shift where we were severely understaffed, responding to a series of high-acuity calls. The relentless pressure, coupled with the emotional toll of witnessing multiple traumatic events, left the entire team exhausted and emotionally drained. That day, we weren't just providing suboptimal patient care; we were putting ourselves and our patients at risk. That experience became a pivotal moment in my commitment to advocating for better working conditions. It highlighted the critical link between our well-being and the quality of care we provide.

This advocacy extends beyond simply complaining about working conditions. It demands a strategic and multi-pronged approach. One of the most effective strategies is unionization. Unions provide a collective voice for paramedics, allowing us to negotiate for better wages, benefits, and working conditions. The power of collective bargaining allows us to address issues that individual paramedics might struggle to tackle alone. Unions can also play a crucial role in ensuring safe working environments, providing legal representation in cases of workplace injury or discrimination, and establishing clear grievance procedures. Joining or strengthening a paramedic union is not just about salary; it's about safeguarding our profession and ensuring our ability to provide effective, safe patient care.

However, unionization isn't a panacea. The effectiveness of a union depends on active participation and strong leadership. Paramedics need to be actively engaged in union activities, attending meetings, participating in negotiations, and holding their union leaders accountable. Apathy and disengagement within the union can undermine its effectiveness, leaving paramedics vulnerable to exploitation and unsafe working conditions. Strong union representation demands a high level of collective action, requiring paramedics to participate in union events and advocate for their colleagues. Furthermore, the effectiveness of unionization can vary depending on the legal and political climate. In certain jurisdictions, the laws governing union activity can make organization and collective bargaining more challenging.

Beyond unionization, political engagement is another critical avenue for advocacy. Paramedics must actively participate in the political process, voting for candidates who support our profession, and lobbying for legislation that protects our interests. This involves educating policymakers about the challenges we face, the importance of our work, and the need for increased funding and resources. It means getting involved in local, state, and national political campaigns, demonstrating the critical role of paramedics within the healthcare system. We must advocate for fair compensation that reflects the complexity and risks inherent in our profession. This involves not just focusing on salary increases but also ensuring adequate benefits packages, including health insurance, retirement plans, and paid time off. These benefits are critical in mitigating the risks of burnout and attracting talented individuals to the field.

Effective advocacy also involves forming strategic alliances with other healthcare organizations and community groups. By building collaborative relationships, we can amplify our voice and build broader support for our concerns. Collaborating with other healthcare professionals, hospital administrators, and community leaders helps create a united front advocating for improvements in pre-hospital care. We can build strong relationships with emergency departments to ensure seamless transitions of patient care, and to advocate for timely and accurate information sharing.

Furthermore, paramedics need to engage in public awareness campaigns to educate the public about the importance of our profession and the challenges we face. This involves sharing our stories, highlighting the demanding nature of our work, and emphasizing the need for better resources and support. By humanizing our profession, we can garner public sympathy and support for our advocacy efforts. This public support can translate to more effective political pressure for improved resources and working conditions. Openly sharing our stories and experiences, both positive and negative, allows the public to understand the demanding nature of the job and to appreciate the value of our service.

We must also focus on improving the image of our profession. The media often portrays paramedics in a sensationalized manner, which can overshadow the true scope and importance of our work. We need to engage in proactive efforts to shape the public narrative surrounding paramedics and to showcase the profound human impact of our jobs. By actively participating in community events, conducting outreach programs, and promoting positive stories, we can work towards a more accurate and realistic depiction of our profession.

Advocating for ourselves isn't about selfishness; it's about ensuring the sustainability of a profession critical to public health. It's about creating a working environment that supports the mental and physical well-being of paramedics, enabling them to provide the high-quality care patients deserve. Our advocacy efforts are directly linked to the safety and well-being of the communities we serve. When we prioritize our own well-being, we ultimately enhance the care we can provide to our patients.

Our advocacy extends far beyond ourselves, impacting the quality of care available to everyone who needs emergency medical services. The investment in our well-being translates to better patient outcomes and a stronger, more sustainable emergency medical services system.

The path to improved working conditions isn't straightforward, but it is essential. It demands persistence, resilience, and a unified approach. By combining strategies like unionization, political engagement, community building, and public awareness campaigns, we can make significant strides toward creating a more supportive, sustainable, and rewarding profession. This isn't just about better pay and benefits; it's about ensuring the future of paramedicine and the well-being of those who dedicate their lives to serving others in their greatest time of need. The fight for improved working conditions is a fight for the future of the profession, and it's a fight we must all be a part of. The legacy of a dedicated paramedic stretches far beyond the immediate scene; it's a legacy of advocating for a profession that so bravely safeguards human life. The fight is far from over, but through unity, persistence, and a shared vision, significant advancements are possible. We owe it to ourselves, our colleagues, and the patients we serve to continue this vital work. Our profession demands our dedication not only to our patients but to ourselves and the future of our colleagues.

The fight for better working conditions and improved patient care extends beyond individual actions and collective bargaining. It necessitates a strategic engagement with professional organizations, forming a crucial network for collaboration and professional growth. These organizations offer a unique platform for paramedics to connect with peers, share experiences, access resources, and collectively advocate for positive change within the profession. My own journey has shown me the power of this interconnectedness. Early in my career, I felt isolated, grappling with the emotional and physical demands of the job, feeling like my struggles were unique. Attending my first national paramedic conference, however, revealed a shared experience; a network of colleagues facing similar challenges, sharing coping strategies, and collectively working toward solutions. That feeling of community and shared purpose was a turning point.

Membership in professional organizations offers a wealth of benefits beyond simple networking. Many organizations provide access to continuing education courses, keeping paramedics updated on the latest advancements in medical techniques, equipment, and emergency protocols. This continuous learning isn't just a matter of maintaining licensure; it's about enhancing the quality of care provided to patients, ensuring that paramedics are equipped to handle the increasingly complex medical scenarios they face daily. I recall a specific instance where a newly introduced cardiac monitoring technique, learned through an organization's online course, proved instrumental in saving a patient's life during a particularly challenging situation. The access to this advanced training, readily available through my professional organization membership, was invaluable.

Beyond educational resources, professional organizations often offer access to liability insurance, a crucial safeguard for paramedics who face significant legal risks in the course of their work. The potential for lawsuits, even in cases of justifiable actions, is ever-present. Having the backing of a robust liability insurance policy, provided through the organization, offers invaluable peace of mind, allowing paramedics to focus on their primary role – providing patient care – without the added burden of financial anxieties related to potential legal disputes. This peace of mind is not simply beneficial for the individual; it contributes to a more confident and effective paramedic workforce.

Furthermore, these organizations frequently lobby for legislative changes that benefit paramedics and the patients they serve. This advocacy work extends beyond the local level, impacting the entire profession at the state and national levels. They work tirelessly to advocate for fair compensation, improved working conditions, increased access to resources, and the establishment of effective regulations that protect both paramedics and the public. I've witnessed firsthand the influence of these organizations in shaping policy decisions impacting ambulance reimbursement rates, staffing levels, and safety protocols. This collective advocacy significantly outweighs the efforts of any individual paramedic striving to create positive change alone.

Active participation within these organizations extends beyond simply receiving benefits; it's about contributing to the professional community. Serving on committees, volunteering for events, or even simply engaging in online discussions allows paramedics to actively shape the direction and priorities of the organization. This direct engagement enables them to influence the agenda, ensuring that the concerns and needs of paramedics at the ground level are heard and addressed effectively. I personally found immense satisfaction in serving on my organization's ethics committee, where we addressed challenging ethical dilemmas faced by paramedics and developed valuable guidelines for decision-making. This collaborative work, impacting the ethical landscape of the entire profession, provided a deeply rewarding and meaningful experience.

Networking opportunities within professional organizations extend beyond simply exchanging contact information. These events facilitate the development of meaningful professional relationships, fostering trust and creating opportunities for mentorship and collaboration. Established paramedics can offer guidance and support to newer members, sharing their experiences and insights, while newer paramedics can bring fresh perspectives and enthusiasm. The cross-generational sharing of knowledge and experience is a cornerstone of professional growth within these organizations, building a strong foundation for the future of the profession. I've benefited significantly from such mentorship relationships throughout my career, receiving valuable advice and support during challenging times.

These organizations often host conferences and workshops that provide opportunities for professional development, beyond the standard continuing education courses. These events provide a chance to learn from leading experts in the field, attend presentations on cutting-edge research, and share experiences with colleagues from across the nation or even internationally. This exposure to diverse perspectives and experiences broadens the horizons of paramedics, strengthening their knowledge base and improving their skills. The access to leading-edge research, presented and discussed at these conferences, has directly impacted my own practice and improved the patient care I provide.

The collaborative spirit fostered within these professional organizations extends to joint advocacy efforts with other healthcare organizations. By forming alliances with hospitals, emergency medical services agencies, and other related groups, paramedics can amplify their advocacy efforts, creating a stronger collective voice for change. These collaborations ensure that paramedics aren't seen as isolated entities, but as integral components of a larger healthcare system, working together to improve the overall quality of patient care. I've witnessed firsthand the success of such collaborations in securing additional funding for EMS services and improving the coordination of care between pre-hospital and in-hospital settings.

Furthermore, the establishment of strong relationships with emergency department physicians and nurses can dramatically improve the efficiency of patient handoffs, ensuring seamless transitions of care and reducing the risk of errors. This collaboration is not merely beneficial for the patient; it directly benefits paramedics by reducing their workload, improving their morale, and increasing their satisfaction with their role within the healthcare continuum. These relationships, built through regular professional interaction and collaborative initiatives, are invaluable to ensuring the efficiency and effectiveness of the entire emergency medical system.

Professional organizations provide a platform for paramedics to engage in research, fostering the advancement of the profession through evidence-based practice. The involvement of paramedics in research initiatives promotes a deeper understanding of the challenges and complexities of pre-hospital care, leading to improvements in both patient outcomes and paramedic well-being. The opportunity to contribute to research, or to simply stay updated on the latest research findings, is an invaluable aspect of professional growth and allows paramedics to engage actively in shaping the future of their profession. Active participation in research, even in a limited capacity, provides a deep sense of fulfillment and contributes to the advancement of knowledge in the field.

In conclusion, professional organizations are not merely professional associations; they are vital components of the paramedic profession, providing invaluable resources, fostering collaboration, facilitating networking, and creating opportunities for professional growth. By actively engaging with these organizations, paramedics can not only improve their own skills and knowledge, but also contribute to the advancement of their profession, enhancing the quality of patient care, and improving the working conditions for all paramedics. The investment in membership and active participation is an investment in the future of paramedicine, a future that demands a united and empowered profession. The benefits are multifaceted, extending from personal professional growth to the broader advancement of pre-hospital emergency care. The collaborative spirit within these organizations provides the essential foundation for continuing to improve the lives of both paramedics and patients alike. This active engagement represents a significant commitment to the profession, enhancing the sustainability and effectiveness of the paramedic service. It is not simply about enhancing individual careers but ensuring the ongoing strength and resilience of the entire profession.

The power to influence policy and practice extends beyond the confines of the ambulance and the emergency department. It requires a proactive approach, a willingness to step outside the immediate demands of daily calls and engage in the broader political and professional landscape. This involves understanding the intricacies of healthcare policy, learning the art of effective advocacy, and building alliances with key stakeholders. It's a challenge, undoubtedly, but one that holds the key to shaping a future where paramedics are valued, respected, and adequately resourced to provide the best possible care.

My own journey into policy advocacy started unexpectedly. A particularly grueling shift, marked by a tragic case involving a delayed response due to inadequate staffing levels, ignited a fire within me. The frustration was palpable, not only for the outcome of the patient's situation, but for the systemic issues that contributed to it. I realized that simply treating patients wasn't enough; I needed to address the root causes of these systemic failures. This realization led me to attend local council meetings, state legislative sessions, and national conferences focused on healthcare reform.

Effective policy advocacy requires understanding the mechanics of policymaking. This involves more than just identifying problems; it necessitates articulating solutions and building support for them. It's about translating the lived experiences of paramedics into tangible policy proposals. It involves researching existing legislation, identifying relevant stakeholders, and crafting persuasive arguments that resonate with policymakers and the public. I learned the hard way that passion alone isn't enough; you need a strategic approach, a well-structured argument, and a thorough understanding of the political process.

One key strategy is to build coalitions. Alone, the voice of a paramedic might be easily dismissed. But united with other professionals – nurses, physicians, hospital administrators, patient advocacy groups – the collective voice becomes powerful, impossible to ignore. I participated in the formation of a coalition to advocate for increased funding for EMS services in our region. We spent months gathering data, presenting evidence of the need for increased resources, and lobbying local government officials. The result was a significant increase in funding, directly impacting staffing levels, equipment upgrades, and improved response times. This success showcased the power of collaborative advocacy.

Another effective strategy is data-driven advocacy. Anecdotal evidence, while compelling, is not always sufficient to sway policymakers. Solid data, meticulously collected and analyzed, provides the weight and credibility necessary to make a real impact. This involves collecting statistics on response times, patient outcomes, and the burden of workplace injuries. This information can then be used to support policy proposals aimed at improving safety, enhancing resource allocation, and improving the overall quality of care. I helped initiate a research project to study the relationship between paramedic burnout and patient safety outcomes. The results demonstrated a clear correlation, which was instrumental in advocating for improved mental health resources for paramedics within our system.

Networking plays a critical role in shaping policy and practice. Building relationships with policymakers, other healthcare professionals, and community leaders creates a network of support that can amplify the influence of paramedics. It involves attending conferences, joining professional organizations, and participating in community events. This networking doesn't just facilitate access to policymakers; it also creates opportunities to learn from others, share experiences, and build a strong base of support. I cultivated strong relationships with several state legislators who were genuinely interested in improving EMS services. These relationships allowed me to provide them with firsthand accounts of the challenges we face, shaping their understanding of the issues and influencing their voting decisions.

Effective communication is the cornerstone of successful policy advocacy. This involves not only clearly articulating the needs and concerns of paramedics but also presenting information in a way that resonates with policymakers and the public. It means tailoring communications to different audiences, utilizing various channels, and maintaining consistent engagement. For instance, we produced a short video showcasing the daily lives of paramedics, highlighting both the rewards and challenges of the profession. This video was distributed through social media, shared with local news outlets, and shown at community events. It humanized the profession and generated widespread support for our policy goals.

Beyond advocating for specific policies, paramedics have a vital role in shaping the broader culture of emergency medical services. This involves promoting professionalism, emphasizing ethical decision-making, and advocating for a culture of continuous learning and improvement. It requires promoting evidence-based practices, participating in professional development activities, and staying abreast of the latest research and advancements. Mentorship is crucial in this process. Experienced paramedics can share their wisdom and expertise with new recruits, shaping the values and practices of the next generation. I have made it a point to mentor new paramedics, encouraging them not only to excel in their technical skills but to become active participants in shaping the future of the profession.

The fight for better working conditions is an integral aspect of shaping policy and practice. This involves advocating for fair compensation, adequate staffing levels, and safe working environments. It requires challenging the status quo, speaking up against injustices, and demanding better protection for paramedics in the face of increasing risks. I witnessed how unsafe working conditions led to burnout and reduced effectiveness. This spurred me to advocate for legislation improving ambulance safety standards and increasing penalties for assaulting emergency personnel.

The challenges are numerous, and the process is often slow and frustrating. Setbacks are inevitable. But the potential rewards are significant. By engaging in policy advocacy, paramedics can create a healthcare system that is better equipped to meet the needs of its citizens, a profession where the individuals who dedicate their lives to saving others are treated with respect and supported with the resources they need to succeed. This doesn't happen by chance; it happens through active engagement and a sustained commitment to making a difference.

This pursuit of a more just and effective system is a marathon, not a sprint. It necessitates resilience, persistence, and a unwavering belief in the importance of our work. There will be days of discouragement, days where progress feels nonexistent. But those days must be viewed not as failures, but as reminders of the ongoing struggle for a more just and effective system. The cumulative effect of sustained effort, of persistent engagement, is transformative. Every small victory, every step forward, builds momentum, creating a stronger foundation for future success.

Ultimately, shaping the future of paramedicine is not solely about enacting specific policies or improving working conditions, but about fostering a culture of continuous improvement and collective responsibility. It's about building a strong, unified professional community dedicated to providing the highest quality patient care within a supportive and sustainable system. It's a journey that requires active participation, creative solutions, and a commitment to making a lasting difference in the lives of both our patients and ourselves. The work is demanding, often frustrating, but the potential to positively impact the lives of countless individuals makes it a worthwhile pursuit. The legacy we leave behind is not measured in individual successes but in the systemic change we create, making the profession we love stronger and more effective for generations to come.

10

Special Populations and Unique Challenges

Pediatric emergencies present a unique set of challenges for paramedics, demanding a different approach than adult care. The seemingly straightforward task of assessing and treating a patient becomes exponentially more complex when that patient is a child. This isn't simply a matter of scaling down adult techniques; it requires a deep understanding of the distinct physiological and developmental nuances of children, as well as the crucial role of communication and family involvement.

One of the most significant differences lies in the physiology of a child. Their smaller size, immature organ systems, and rapid metabolic rate dramatically alter how they respond to illness or injury. For instance, a child's airway is proportionally smaller and more easily obstructed than an adult's. A seemingly minor swelling can rapidly compromise their breathing, requiring immediate intervention. Their relatively higher surface area to body mass ratio makes them more susceptible to hypothermia, while their immature immune systems leave them vulnerable to infection. A seemingly minor cut can lead to a severe infection in a child more readily than in an adult, necessitating careful wound management and prompt antibiotic administration when indicated. Dehydration is also a major concern; children can become severely dehydrated quickly, leading to potentially life-threatening complications. I remember a call involving a toddler who had been vomiting and had diarrhea for 24 hours. He presented with significant signs of dehydration, including sunken eyes and decreased skin turgor. Rapid fluid resuscitation was critical, and it highlighted the rapid deterioration children can experience.

Furthermore, children's responses to trauma differ significantly from adults. Their bones are more flexible, making fractures less obvious initially. Internal injuries might not present with the same clear signs as in adults. A child who has fallen from a height might seem superficially uninjured, but could be suffering from internal bleeding or a head injury. This necessitates a thorough and systematic assessment, looking beyond the immediately visible signs of injury. I once responded to a call where a child had fallen from a tree. The initial assessment revealed only minor scrapes and bruises. However, persistent questioning of the child and their parents revealed subtle changes in behavior and alertness. Further investigation in the emergency department uncovered a significant concussion that could have easily been missed without a meticulous approach.

Effective communication is paramount in pediatric emergencies. Unlike adults who can often articulate their symptoms and concerns, children may not be able to communicate their discomfort or the nature of their illness. This necessitates relying on observation, understanding nonverbal cues, and involving the child's parents or guardians. Parents are an invaluable resource, providing crucial information about the child's medical history, allergies, and any previous illnesses. Their presence often provides comfort and reassurance to the child, reducing anxiety and improving cooperation during examination and treatment. However, it's also important to remember that parents may be overwhelmed by the situation and their own anxieties, requiring sensitive and empathetic communication from the paramedic team.

One of the most challenging aspects of pediatric emergency care is managing a child's anxiety and fear. The emergency setting can be overwhelming for a child, and their fear can interfere with the assessment and treatment process. Using age-appropriate language, offering choices when possible (e.g., "Would you like to sit here or lie down?"), maintaining a calm and reassuring demeanor, and involving the child in the process whenever feasible are crucial strategies. I recall attending to a young girl who had suffered a minor burn. Instead of simply applying the dressing, I showed her the antiseptic wipes and explained what I was doing, making the process less frightening and more collaborative. This small act of involving her fostered trust and cooperation.

Different age groups require different approaches. Infants may need more specialized care, requiring knowledge of their unique physiology and vulnerabilities. Toddlers and preschoolers may be more easily distracted, requiring creative techniques to assess them. School-aged children can often provide more detailed information about their symptoms, but may still need reassurance and support. Adolescents often present with unique challenges, especially around privacy and autonomy. This requires navigating complex issues of consent and confidentiality while ensuring they receive appropriate medical attention. Each age group presents distinct communication challenges, highlighting the importance of tailoring our approach to the individual child's developmental stage.

The assessment of a child in an emergency situation requires a structured and systematic approach. The ABCs (airway, breathing, circulation) remain paramount, but the assessment should also consider the child's overall appearance, level of consciousness, and response to stimuli. While adult assessments often rely heavily on verbal responses, pediatric assessments necessitate a keen eye for subtle signs of distress, such as changes in respiratory rate, skin color, and level of activity. We need to be astute observers, recognizing subtle changes that may indicate a serious underlying condition. I remember a case where a young child appeared lethargic and withdrawn, initially presenting as simply tired. However, upon closer observation, I noticed subtle changes in his breathing pattern and skin color, leading to a more thorough assessment that revealed a severe infection.

Treating children requires a precise and calculated approach, often employing age-appropriate dosages and techniques. Medications need to be carefully calculated based on weight and body surface area, considering their potential side effects and interactions with other medications. Intravenous access can be challenging in children, requiring specialized techniques and understanding of their delicate vascular systems. I've found that establishing rapport and distraction techniques are often essential in securing IV access successfully. The use of non-pharmacological methods of pain relief, such as distraction, positioning, and comfort measures, is especially important in pediatric care, minimizing the need for sedation or analgesia whenever possible.

Ethical considerations are often heightened in pediatric emergencies. Parental consent is typically required for treatment, but in situations where the child's life is at immediate risk, actions may need to be taken before consent is obtained. Balancing the child's best interests with parental wishes can create ethically complex situations, requiring careful consideration and a clear understanding of relevant legal guidelines. Navigating these situations requires both professional expertise and emotional intelligence, demanding a delicate balance between respecting parental rights and prioritizing the child's safety and well-being. It requires a deep understanding of ethical principles and a willingness to advocate for the child's best interests.

Beyond the immediate medical care, the paramedic's role extends to supporting the family during this stressful time. Providing clear and concise information, answering their questions honestly and compassionately, and offering emotional support are crucial components of providing holistic care. This can involve coordinating with the emergency department staff, ensuring a smooth transition of care and providing updates to the family throughout the process. I found that simply being present, offering a listening ear, and showing genuine empathy can make a profound difference in a family's experience during a challenging time.

In conclusion, pediatric emergencies pose unique challenges that require specialized knowledge, skills, and a profound understanding of child development and family dynamics. Paramedics involved in pediatric care must be adept at adapting their techniques, communication styles, and ethical decision-making processes to meet the specific needs of this vulnerable population. It's a demanding yet profoundly rewarding aspect of paramedicine, emphasizing the importance of constant learning, rigorous self-reflection, and an unwavering commitment to providing compassionate and effective care for the youngest among our patients. The combination of advanced medical knowledge and empathetic engagement is what truly defines success in pediatric emergency medicine.

Geriatric emergencies demand a fundamentally different approach than those involving younger adults. The complexities introduced by age-related physiological changes, comorbidities, and the often-fragile social support systems of older adults necessitate a heightened level of awareness, patience, and clinical acumen. It's a realm of paramedicine that requires a nuanced understanding beyond simply applying standard protocols, demanding instead a tailored approach born from experience and empathy.

One of the most striking differences lies in the often-blurred presentation of symptoms. What might be a straightforward myocardial infarction in a younger patient can manifest subtly, with atypical chest pain, shortness of breath, or even just generalized weakness in an older adult. Their sensory impairments, such as diminished hearing or vision, can further complicate the assessment process, hindering effective communication and potentially delaying diagnosis. I vividly remember a call involving an elderly woman who presented with confusion and a slight fall. Initially, it seemed like a simple syncopal episode. However, upon closer questioning (and employing a large-print communication card!), we discovered she had been experiencing subtle chest discomfort for days. Further investigation revealed a significant cardiac event that had been masked by her age-related changes and diminished communication capabilities.

Polypharmacy is a pervasive issue in geriatric patients, presenting significant challenges in medication reconciliation and treatment decisions. Many older adults take numerous medications to manage various chronic conditions, increasing the risk of drug interactions and adverse effects. Understanding a patient's entire medication regimen is crucial in determining the cause of their emergency, preventing dangerous drug interactions, and ensuring safe medication administration. One seemingly minor detail – a missed dose of a blood thinner or an interaction between two commonly prescribed medications – could dramatically alter the patient's condition and complicate our treatment strategy. On one call, we encountered an elderly gentleman suffering from severe gastrointestinal bleeding. After a painstaking review of his numerous medications, we discovered an interaction between two drugs he was taking that had significantly increased his risk of bleeding. This highlighted the importance of meticulous medication review in every geriatric emergency.

Furthermore, the prevalence of chronic conditions in this population significantly impacts emergency response. Conditions such as heart failure, chronic obstructive pulmonary disease (COPD), diabetes, and dementia are common among the elderly, often coexisting and complicating both assessment and treatment. A seemingly straightforward respiratory distress call might be rooted in a COPD exacerbation complicated by heart failure, requiring a multifaceted approach involving oxygen therapy, fluid management, and potentially medications to address both conditions concurrently. The interplay of these comorbidities can create a complex clinical picture, demanding a thorough understanding of the individual patient's medical history and a well-coordinated response.

Age-related physiological changes also play a significant role in shaping our response. Reduced cardiac reserve, decreased lung capacity, and altered thermoregulation can all influence how an older adult reacts to illness or injury. What might be a manageable injury in a younger person can lead to a life-threatening situation in an older adult. A simple fall, for instance, could result in a hip fracture, a significant event with potential for life-threatening complications. Their reduced physiological reserves mean they often compensate less effectively for injuries or illnesses. We need to anticipate this reduced physiological reserve, making quicker assessments, prioritising rapid interventions and initiating transport more decisively than we might with a younger patient.

Effective communication with geriatric patients requires an approach built on patience and understanding. Hearing and vision impairments are common, demanding clear and concise communication, perhaps using visual aids or written communication where appropriate. Cognitive impairment, such as dementia, can further complicate communication, requiring us to involve family members or caregivers whenever possible. Building trust and rapport is paramount; a calm and reassuring demeanor can significantly improve cooperation during the assessment and treatment. In several cases, I found that simply taking the time to establish a connection, speaking slowly and clearly, and demonstrating patience can significantly improve communication with a patient who initially seemed agitated and confused. Listening attentively and respecting their autonomy, even in situations of diminished cognitive capacity, is critical.

The physical examination of an older adult needs to be adapted to their physical limitations. We need to be mindful of their potential fragility and adjust our handling accordingly. Their skin is often more fragile, making careful palpation essential to avoid bruising or tearing. Their decreased mobility might necessitate additional support during the examination. I've learned to be extremely careful in moving older adults, using appropriate lifting techniques and additional support personnel when necessary. This not only minimizes the risk of additional injuries but also demonstrates respect and empathy.

Furthermore, the social support network of the patient needs to be considered. Older adults often rely on family members, friends, or caregivers for support. Assessing their support system is crucial for planning discharge and ensuring their safe transition back to their home environment. Determining who's responsible for their care, their living situation, and their ability to cope with their ongoing needs can be critical to ensure appropriate referral to social services or other supportive systems. We're not just treating the immediate emergency; we're a key part of a larger care continuum.

Finally, ethical considerations become even more prominent in geriatric emergencies. Advance directives, such as Do Not Resuscitate (DNR) orders, are frequently encountered in this population. Respecting these directives is paramount, ensuring that patient autonomy is upheld and their wishes are honored. However, it's also crucial to thoroughly assess the circumstances, considering the specific situation and whether the current presentation aligns with the patient's previously expressed wishes. Balancing patient autonomy with the responsibility to provide life-saving intervention requires careful consideration, sound clinical judgment, and a deep understanding of legal and ethical guidelines. It's often a delicate balance between respecting their wishes and ensuring their comfort, a balancing act I've repeatedly found requires significant reflective consideration.

In conclusion, geriatric emergencies require a specialized approach, demanding both advanced medical knowledge and an empathetic understanding of the unique challenges posed by aging. It calls for a detailed assessment, effective communication strategies, consideration of co-morbidities and polypharmacy, sensitivity to physical limitations, and careful respect for patient autonomy. It's a complex area of paramedic practice, but one that is profoundly rewarding when we successfully navigate these challenges and provide compassionate, effective care for our aging patients. The experience requires a constant reflection on our approaches, an ongoing learning journey designed to improve our efficacy and understanding of this vulnerable and valuable population.

Behavioral health emergencies represent a significant and growing portion of our workload. Unlike many physical emergencies where the diagnosis is often relatively clear-cut, behavioral health crises present a complex and often unpredictable challenge. The lack of readily apparent physical pathology initially can make these calls deceptively straightforward. Yet, the potential for violence, self-harm, or sudden decompensation demands a measured, patient, and highly skilled approach. It's a realm where technical proficiency alone is insufficient; empathy, active listening, and a deep understanding of human behavior become paramount.

My first encounter with a truly significant behavioral health emergency came early in my career. A young man, barely out of his teens, was barricaded inside his apartment, armed with a knife, and threatening self-harm. The scene was tense, the air thick with the unspoken fear of those gathered outside. The police were present, forming a perimeter, and the pressure was immense. My training kicked in, but it felt inadequate against the raw, volatile energy emanating from the apartment.

Our role wasn't to subdue him; it was to assess his condition, understand his distress, and facilitate a safe resolution. Hours were spent communicating through the door, building rapport, offering reassurance, and gently coaxing him towards surrender. It was exhausting, both emotionally and mentally. But when he finally emerged, his tears a testament to his pain and our perseverance, it solidified my understanding of this critical facet of paramedicine. It's a victory not of force, but of patience, empathy, and a deep understanding of the underlying crisis.

Successful management of behavioral health emergencies hinges on a thorough and careful assessment. However, unlike a physical trauma, the "vitals" are less tangible. Instead of blood pressure and heart rate, we are looking for behavioral cues – agitation, anxiety, paranoia, or depression. It's about listening for the unspoken pain, understanding the nuances of body language, and recognizing the triggers that might escalate the situation. This requires a non-judgmental approach, creating a safe space for the individual to express their feelings and concerns. We need to remember that people in crisis are not acting rationally; their behavior is often a manifestation of their internal turmoil.

De-escalation is the cornerstone of our intervention. It's a gradual process, not a forceful takedown. It begins with establishing a calm and reassuring presence, using a quiet, respectful tone of voice. Maintaining eye contact, but without being intrusive, can build trust. Employing active listening techniques, repeating back what they've said to confirm understanding, shows that we're genuinely listening to their concerns. Understanding their immediate needs and stressors is paramount. Are they hungry? Tired? Are they experiencing hallucinations or delusions? Addressing these immediate physical and psychological needs can often pave the way for de-escalation.

Physical space plays a crucial role. We must maintain a safe distance, avoiding any gestures or actions that might be misinterpreted as threatening. Our body language should reflect calm assurance, not fear or aggression. Often, even small adjustments, such as lowering the tone of our voice or slightly shifting our stance, can diffuse tension. One technique I've found effective is to mirror the patient's posture subtly; it creates a subconscious connection and promotes a sense of understanding and rapport. This might seem like a small detail, but it's often the subtle nuances that make the difference in crisis situations.

Communication is key, but it's not just about what we say; it's about how we say it. Simple, clear language, avoiding jargon or technical terms, is crucial. We should always validate their feelings, even if we don't necessarily agree with their perspective. A phrase as simple as, "I can see you're feeling really upset right now," can be profoundly validating. Reassurance is equally important. We might assure them that help is available, that we're there to support them, and that things will get better.

In many cases, involving family members or caregivers can be crucial. If the individual has a support network, their presence can often provide comfort and reassurance, facilitating a smoother de-escalation process. However, this involvement must be handled carefully, respecting the individual's wishes and maintaining their autonomy. Their perspective can also provide invaluable insight into the individual's history, triggers, and current state of mind. Furthermore, their assistance in medication reconciliation can prevent potentially adverse interactions, ensuring the safety and well-being of the patient.

Sometimes, despite our best efforts, de-escalation isn't possible. We must always prioritize safety, both our own and the patient's. If the individual becomes violent or poses a threat to themselves or others, we may need to employ restraints, but only as a last resort, and always with the appropriate level of force and under the guidance of law enforcement. Documentation is critical in these situations, detailing our actions, the reason for restraint, and the individual's response. It's a delicate balance between ensuring safety and avoiding unnecessary escalation, a fine line that can easily be crossed without careful consideration.

Once the situation is stabilized, our role shifts to ensuring appropriate transfer to a mental health facility. This often involves coordinating with law enforcement, mental health professionals, and family members. The transition should be handled sensitively, with dignity and respect for the individual's privacy and autonomy. The key is not to abandon them but to facilitate a safe and supportive transfer to a setting where they can receive the appropriate level of care.

The emotional toll of dealing with behavioral health emergencies cannot be understated. These are emotionally draining calls, leaving us confronting human vulnerability and despair. We're witnessing pain, often in its rawest form. It's crucial to process these experiences; we can't simply compartmentalize them and move on. Self-care, peer support, and seeking professional help when needed are essential to prevent burnout and moral injury. These calls are taxing, and recognizing the importance of aftercare is just as crucial as the immediate intervention. Our ability to handle these complex situations with empathy, patience, and skill directly impacts our own well-being.

In conclusion, managing behavioral health emergencies is a complex but vital aspect of paramedicine. It demands a multifaceted approach integrating de-escalation techniques, active listening, clear communication, and careful attention to safety. It requires patience, empathy, and a profound understanding of human behavior. The ability to build rapport, validate feelings, and facilitate a safe transition to appropriate care sets skilled paramedics apart in these challenging, and increasingly prevalent, situations. It's a testament to the crucial role we play in the larger healthcare system, going beyond the technical skills and embracing the human element of care. The ongoing reflection on our approach, the debriefings with colleagues, and the constant pursuit of better training are what ultimately ensure that we are providing not just treatment, but genuine compassion in our interactions with those in behavioral health crisis. Our responsibility extends beyond simply stabilizing the patient's condition; it encompasses their emotional well-being and their pathway toward recovery.

Trauma in vulnerable populations presents a complex interplay of social determinants, healthcare access, and individual experiences, often resulting in disparities in the quality and timeliness of care. These disparities aren't simply statistical anomalies; they represent a systemic failure to address the unique needs of individuals and communities facing significant social, economic, and health-related challenges. My experience has shown me that while the physiological aspects of trauma care remain constant, the social context profoundly influences how we approach, treat, and ultimately, support the recovery of these patients.

One of the most striking disparities lies in access to pre-hospital care. Individuals living in underserved communities, often characterized by poverty, limited transportation, and a lack of adequate infrastructure, frequently experience longer response times and delayed access to emergency medical services. This delay, even a matter of minutes, can be catastrophic in trauma situations, impacting survival rates and long-term outcomes. I recall a call to a rural community where a severe motor vehicle accident had occurred. The nearest trauma center was an hour's drive away, a journey significantly prolonged by the winding, poorly maintained roads. The delay in reaching definitive care, compounded by the challenges of transporting the critically injured patient across difficult terrain, underscored the stark reality of geographic disparities in access to timely trauma care.

Beyond geographical limitations, socioeconomic factors contribute significantly to disparities in trauma care. Patients from low-income backgrounds often face barriers to accessing appropriate follow-up care, including rehabilitation services, medication, and ongoing medical monitoring. The financial burden of medical expenses, coupled with the potential loss of income due to injury or disability, can further exacerbate their vulnerability. I've witnessed firsthand the struggle of families grappling with both the immediate trauma and the long-term financial repercussions, often leading to compromised adherence to treatment plans and potentially poorer outcomes. This financial strain, frequently overlooked in the immediate aftermath of a traumatic incident, can cast a long shadow on the recovery process.

Cultural competency plays a crucial role in bridging the gap in trauma care for vulnerable populations. Effective communication, sensitivity to cultural beliefs and practices, and an understanding of diverse health literacy levels are essential in building trust and ensuring the provision of culturally appropriate care. Language barriers can create significant obstacles, impeding effective communication during assessment, treatment, and the crucial transfer of information to other healthcare providers. A significant portion of our population relies on language access services, and ensuring sufficient access to interpreters remains a key challenge. On one occasion, I responded to a call involving a family who primarily spoke Spanish. Their understandable anxiety was compounded by the difficulty in communication. With the help of a bilingual colleague and a telephone translation service, we were able to achieve a degree of understanding and provide appropriate care, but the incident highlighted the difficulties posed by language differences in emergency situations and the importance of investing in proper training and culturally competent staff.

Furthermore, trauma care must acknowledge and actively address the impact of systemic racism and discrimination. Studies have consistently shown that racial and ethnic minorities often experience disparities in access to and quality of healthcare, including trauma care. These disparities may stem from implicit biases, unequal access to resources, and historical and ongoing systemic inequities. Addressing these systemic issues necessitates a concerted effort towards comprehensive system reform, including improving access to healthcare, addressing social determinants of health, and promoting culturally competent healthcare practices.

The unique challenges faced by vulnerable populations in trauma care extend beyond physical injuries. Individuals experiencing homelessness, those with mental health conditions, and those from marginalized communities often have complex medical and social needs that necessitate a more holistic and integrated approach to care. These populations may face greater barriers to accessing healthcare in general, may have pre-existing conditions that complicate injury management, and may be more likely to experience secondary trauma, such as social isolation and economic instability. They often lack the same support systems that assist in recovery from traumatic injuries.

Addressing these disparities demands a multifaceted approach that goes beyond individual interventions. This includes implementing proactive measures to improve access to healthcare services, investing in culturally competent and trauma-informed care, advocating for policies that address the social determinants of health, and fostering community partnerships to improve health equity. As paramedics, we are on the front lines of this challenge, and our role extends beyond simply providing emergency medical care. We are frequently the first point of contact for many patients and are in a unique position to assess needs, advocate for support, and help bridge the gap to long-term care.

The mental health consequences of trauma are often profound and should not be overlooked, especially within vulnerable populations. Trauma can exacerbate pre-existing mental health conditions, leading to increased rates of depression, anxiety, PTSD, and substance use disorders. Furthermore, the social and economic consequences of trauma, such as job loss and housing instability, can further contribute to mental health challenges. We need to provide not only physical trauma care but also readily accessible mental health support systems, early intervention strategies, and tailored mental health resources designed to meet the diverse needs of these populations.

In conclusion, ensuring equitable access to trauma care for vulnerable populations requires a fundamental shift in how we approach emergency medical services and healthcare in general. It necessitates a commitment to addressing the social determinants of health, investing in culturally competent and trauma-informed care, and implementing systemic changes to address disparities in access to and quality of healthcare. Our role as paramedics is not simply to treat the immediate physical injuries; it's also to advocate for our patients, acknowledge their experiences, and work towards creating a healthcare system that is truly equitable and just. As we reflect on the diverse challenges faced by our patients, we must recommit to providing comprehensive, empathetic, and culturally sensitive care that meets the unique needs of each individual, promoting not just their physical healing, but their overall well-being and recovery. This means acknowledging the systemic factors contributing to health inequities and striving towards a more just and equitable healthcare system for all. The task is not simple; but the ethical imperative to address these disparities in our profession is profound.

Obstetric emergencies present a unique and often high-stakes challenge for paramedics. Unlike many other emergencies where the immediate threat is often readily apparent, obstetric calls demand a nuanced understanding of physiological changes, potential complications, and the emotional and psychological aspects of pregnancy and childbirth. This isn't simply about managing a medical crisis; it's about navigating a deeply personal and often vulnerable moment in a woman's life, requiring a high degree of empathy and sensitivity alongside our technical expertise.

One of the most critical aspects of obstetric emergency care is accurate and timely assessment. The initial moments on scene are crucial for identifying potential complications. This involves quickly assessing the mother's vital signs, determining the gestational age, evaluating the frequency and intensity of contractions, and checking for signs of vaginal bleeding, fetal distress, or pre-eclampsia. We use a systematic approach, incorporating our knowledge of normal physiological changes during pregnancy and labor, while remaining vigilant for deviations from the norm. I remember a call involving a young woman in her late stages of pregnancy who presented with sudden, severe abdominal pain. Initially, we suspected appendicitis, a common differential diagnosis. However, a closer examination revealed subtle signs of placental abruption, a life-threatening condition requiring immediate intervention. This highlighted the importance of maintaining a broad differential diagnosis, considering the complexities of pregnancy, and remaining open to the unexpected.

Pre-eclampsia, characterized by high blood pressure and protein in the urine, represents a significant threat to both mother and fetus. Recognizing the warning signs—such as severe headache, visual disturbances, and swelling—is vital for early intervention. Delayed recognition and treatment can lead to eclampsia, a life-threatening condition involving seizures, further complicating the situation and increasing the risk of maternal and fetal mortality. Our training emphasizes the recognition of pre-eclampsia and prompt transport to a facility equipped to manage this condition, often involving specialized obstetric care units.

Another critical area is the management of postpartum hemorrhage (PPH). PPH is a leading cause of maternal mortality worldwide, and prompt intervention is crucial. This involves controlling bleeding through various techniques, including uterine massage, administering uterotonic medications, and, in severe cases, surgical intervention. However, managing PPH is about more than just technical skill; it requires a calm and organized approach, as the emotional distress of the mother, and those around her, can quickly escalate in these stressful situations. I remember a case where a young mother experienced severe PPH immediately after delivery. The sheer volume of blood loss was alarming, and the scene was fraught with emotion. Through careful coordination with the emergency room team and a clear, organized approach, we were able to stabilize the patient and get her to the hospital in time for life-saving intervention. The experience underscored the importance of teamwork, clear communication, and maintaining composure under immense pressure.

Fetal distress presents a similarly complex and time-sensitive challenge. Monitoring fetal heart rate, assessing the mother's condition, and recognizing signs of placental insufficiency or umbilical cord compression are all essential for effective intervention. In situations of prolonged fetal distress, the decision to perform an emergency cesarean section en route to the hospital may be necessary. Of course, only specially trained paramedics are equipped to execute such critical procedures. This involves a thorough understanding of the potential risks and benefits of on-scene interventions, including the limitations of pre-hospital care, and collaboration with the receiving hospital.

The management of ectopic pregnancies highlights the subtle yet critical nature of obstetric emergencies. Ectopic pregnancies, where the fertilized egg implants outside the uterus, can cause internal bleeding and require immediate surgical intervention. Recognizing the subtle signs of ectopic pregnancy, such as abdominal pain, vaginal bleeding, and amenorrhea, can be challenging, especially in early stages. Paramedics play a vital role in ensuring early detection and timely transport to an appropriate facility, where definitive diagnosis and treatment can be provided. Early recognition can often be the difference between a successful outcome and a life-threatening emergency.

Providing care during obstetric emergencies is far from a solo endeavor. It necessitates effective teamwork and interprofessional collaboration. Clear communication with emergency medical dispatch, emergency room staff, and the hospital's obstetric team is paramount for ensuring a coordinated and successful outcome. The seamless transfer of information, including the mother's medical history, vital signs, and any interventions performed, is crucial for ensuring continuity of care. This collaborative spirit underscores the collective responsibility we have in ensuring safe and effective care, especially given the high stakes involved in these situations.

The emotional toll on both the patient and the care provider must not be underestimated. Pregnancy and childbirth are inherently emotional experiences, and emergencies heighten the level of anxiety and stress significantly. Paramedics need to be sensitive to these emotional dimensions and provide compassionate and supportive care. This might involve offering reassurance, providing information about the situation and the plan of care, and creating a safe and supportive environment for the patient. As paramedics, our roles often extend beyond the purely medical; we become support systems, offering empathy and understanding at moments of significant vulnerability and fear. Maintaining this emotional equilibrium can be exhausting, but it is a necessary component of providing truly comprehensive care.

Furthermore, continuing education and regular training are essential for paramedics involved in obstetric emergencies. Advanced life support training, focused obstetric courses, and simulation scenarios are crucial for maintaining competency and adapting to advancements in medical knowledge and technology. The rapidly evolving nature of medical science, coupled with the complexity of obstetric emergencies, demands an ongoing commitment to professional development.

In conclusion, providing care during pregnancy and delivery presents a unique set of challenges and requires a specialized skill set. The ability to accurately assess the situation, recognize life-threatening complications, and effectively manage them demands both extensive knowledge and exceptional judgment. But above all, it requires empathy and understanding, acknowledging the deeply personal nature of these moments in a woman's life. Collaboration and teamwork are essential, and the emotional toll on the care providers should not be minimized. In this demanding aspect of our profession, the dedication to continuous learning, and a commitment to compassionate care, is paramount in ensuring the well-being of both the mother and child. This commitment, fueled by professional experience and a compassionate heart, serves as the foundation of truly effective and empathetic paramedic practice.

11

The Science of Paramedicine

The human body is a remarkably resilient machine, capable of incredible feats of adaptation and survival. Yet, this same resilience is tested to its limits during emergencies. Understanding the physiological and pathophysiological responses to trauma and illness is fundamental to effective paramedic practice. It allows us to anticipate complications, make informed clinical decisions, and ultimately, improve patient outcomes. This section will explore the body's stress response, focusing on key systems and their vulnerabilities in emergency situations.

One of the most fundamental responses to stress is the activation of the sympathetic nervous system, often referred to as the "fight-or-flight" response. This ancient mechanism, honed over millennia of evolutionary pressure, prepares the body for immediate action. The release of adrenaline and noradrenaline leads to a cascade of effects: increased heart rate and blood pressure, dilated pupils, and shunting of blood away from non-essential organs to the brain, heart, and muscles. While beneficial in the face of immediate danger, a prolonged or overly intense sympathetic response can be detrimental. The sustained elevation of blood pressure can strain the cardiovascular system, potentially leading to myocardial ischemia or even infarction. The diversion of blood flow can compromise organ function, particularly in the kidneys and gastrointestinal tract.

I vividly recall a call involving a young man involved in a high-speed motorcycle accident. On arrival, he was in obvious distress, exhibiting signs of significant blood loss and respiratory compromise. His heart was racing, his blood pressure was dangerously high, and his breathing was shallow and rapid. The sympathetic nervous system was clearly in overdrive. While we focused on stabilizing his airway and controlling the bleeding, we were acutely aware of the potential for cardiac complications. The rapid heart rate, coupled with the stress on his circulatory system, put him at significant risk of a cardiac event. It's in such moments that the fundamental understanding of physiology allows for strategic management. We chose to administer fluids carefully, monitoring his vital signs meticulously, and ensured rapid transport to the trauma center. His successful recovery, albeit a close call, reinforced the importance of understanding the body's response to severe trauma.

Beyond the sympathetic nervous system, the endocrine system plays a significant role in the stress response. The release of cortisol, a glucocorticoid hormone, influences numerous metabolic processes, providing a sustained energy supply for the body's needs. Cortisol raises blood glucose levels, increases protein breakdown, and suppresses the immune system. While beneficial in the short term, chronic elevation of cortisol can lead to immunosuppression, making the individual more susceptible to infection. Prolonged stress also negatively impacts the gastrointestinal tract, causing issues such as nausea, vomiting, and diarrhea. Moreover, chronic exposure to elevated cortisol levels is associated with a range of adverse health effects, including increased risk of cardiovascular disease, obesity, and mood disorders.

The respiratory system is another crucial component of the body's stress response. During emergencies, the body's demand for oxygen increases significantly. The respiratory rate and depth increase to meet this heightened demand. However, various factors can compromise respiratory function in an emergency setting. Trauma to the chest wall, for example, can cause rib fractures and pneumothorax, leading to impaired ventilation and hypoxia. Additionally, airway obstruction, whether due to foreign bodies, swelling, or other factors, can severely restrict oxygen uptake. As paramedics, we must quickly recognize and address any respiratory compromise, ensuring adequate oxygenation through interventions such as airway management, supplemental oxygen administration, and mechanical ventilation where necessary.

One case that stands out involved a patient experiencing anaphylactic shock following a bee sting. The rapid onset of respiratory distress, characterized by wheezing and shortness of breath, necessitated immediate intervention. We promptly administered epinephrine, a potent bronchodilator and vasoconstrictor, while simultaneously providing high-flow oxygen. The immediate improvement in the patient's respiratory status highlighted the importance of a swift and targeted response to acute respiratory emergencies. This situation underscores the interconnectedness of physiological systems and how a seemingly isolated event can rapidly affect multiple body systems.

The cardiovascular system, the body's circulatory network, is profoundly affected by stress. Increased heart rate and blood pressure, driven by the sympathetic nervous system, increase the workload on the heart. In individuals with pre-existing cardiovascular conditions, this increased demand can exacerbate underlying issues, leading to angina, myocardial infarction, or even cardiac arrest. Furthermore, blood loss, as seen in trauma cases, can rapidly lead to hypovolemic shock, a life-threatening condition characterized by inadequate tissue perfusion. Prompt fluid resuscitation and blood product administration are crucial in managing hypovolemic shock, but they can be complex to deliver pre-hospital and require meticulous monitoring to prevent complications.

The kidneys, essential for maintaining fluid and electrolyte balance, are susceptible to damage during emergencies. Hypoperfusion, often associated with shock, can impair renal function, potentially leading to acute kidney injury. The use of nephrotoxic drugs, combined with conditions like hypovolemia, can further stress these critical organs. In certain cases, rhabdomyolysis – breakdown of muscle tissue releasing damaging substances into the bloodstream – can lead to acute renal failure requiring extensive hospital care.

The neurological system, responsible for coordinating all body functions, is acutely vulnerable in emergencies. Traumatic brain injury (TBI), a common finding in high-impact collisions, can have devastating consequences. Even subtle neurological changes, such as altered mental status or focal neurological deficits, can indicate underlying brain damage, highlighting the need for careful neurological assessment and timely intervention. Stroke, a sudden disruption of blood flow to the brain, presents a unique set of challenges, necessitating rapid identification and management to minimize long-term neurological damage. The time-sensitive nature of stroke treatment emphasizes the crucial role of rapid assessment and efficient transportation to appropriate healthcare facilities. I have encountered several stroke cases where early recognition and immediate transport to a stroke center were instrumental in preserving neurological function.

The integumentary system, encompassing the skin, plays a vital role in maintaining thermoregulation and protecting against infection. Significant injuries to the skin can compromise this protective barrier, resulting in fluid loss, hypothermia, and increased susceptibility to infection. Burns, particularly severe burns, can lead to substantial fluid shifts, posing a significant challenge to fluid management. Extensive burns create a significant challenge in maintaining fluid balance and preventing hypovolemic shock. Our understanding of fluid dynamics, burn physiology, and the complications of burn injuries is crucial in providing effective prehospital care.

The gastrointestinal system, while often overlooked in acute emergency scenarios, can be significantly affected. Stress-induced nausea, vomiting, and diarrhea are common. More serious issues, like internal bleeding or organ damage, can also occur, necessitating close monitoring and appropriate intervention. Our role, beyond immediate life-saving measures, extends to assessing and managing the potential for GI complications resulting from stress or direct trauma.

The immune system, a complex network responsible for defending against infection, is often suppressed during periods of prolonged or severe stress. This increased vulnerability underscores the importance of infection control and preventive measures, especially in situations involving trauma and significant physiological insult.

In summary, understanding the interplay between these physiological systems during emergencies is paramount for effective paramedic practice. Recognizing the body's stress response, anticipating potential complications, and providing timely and appropriate interventions are critical in improving patient outcomes. This deep understanding of the science underpinning our work empowers us to make informed decisions under pressure, navigating the complexities of human physiology in moments of crisis. The relentless pursuit of knowledge, coupled with hands-on experience, forms the backbone of a competent and compassionate paramedic.

Building upon our understanding of the intricate physiological responses to trauma and illness, we now delve into the crucial role of pharmacology in paramedicine. This is not merely about memorizing drug names and dosages; it's about grasping the fundamental mechanisms by which these medications interact with the human body, influencing its delicate balance to alleviate suffering and potentially save lives. The effective and safe administration of medications is a cornerstone of our practice, requiring not only knowledge but also a deep appreciation for the potential benefits and risks involved.

Let's begin with the foundational concept of pharmacodynamics – how a drug affects the body. This involves understanding the drug's mechanism of action: how it interacts with receptors, enzymes, or other cellular components to produce its therapeutic effect. For instance, consider morphine, a powerful opioid analgesic. It acts by binding to opioid receptors in the central nervous system, reducing the perception of pain. This is a relatively straightforward mechanism, but the nuances are critical. Different opioid receptors respond with varying intensity to morphine, leading to a range of effects, from analgesia to respiratory depression. This understanding is vital because it helps us anticipate potential side effects and adjust our treatment accordingly. A patient's age, weight, and underlying medical conditions significantly influence how they respond to medication. This calls for careful consideration before administering any drug, emphasizing the need for accurate assessment and individualized treatment plans.

Pharmacokinetics, on the other hand, describes what the body does to the drug. This encompasses absorption, distribution, metabolism, and excretion – the four processes that govern a drug's journey through the body. Absorption refers to how the drug enters the bloodstream. The route of administration plays a crucial role here: intravenous medications enter the bloodstream immediately, while oral medications undergo absorption in the gastrointestinal tract, a process that can be variable depending on factors like gastric emptying and gut motility. Distribution describes how the drug spreads throughout the body, reaching its target sites and other tissues. Factors such as blood flow, protein binding, and the drug's lipid solubility determine how effectively it is distributed. Metabolism, primarily in the liver, involves the chemical modification of the drug, often converting it into a less active or inactive form. Finally, excretion, primarily through the kidneys, removes the drug and its metabolites from the body. Understanding these processes allows us to predict how long a drug's effects will last and to anticipate potential drug interactions. For example, a patient with com-

promised liver function may require a lower dose of a medication exten-
sively metabolized by the liver to prevent toxicity.

Consider the administration of naloxone, an opioid antagonist, to
a patient experiencing an opioid overdose. Understanding the pharmacokinetics of both naloxone and the opioid helps determine the appropriate dose and route of administration. Naloxone's rapid onset of
action, achieved through intravenous administration, is crucial in these
life-threatening situations. Its relatively short half-life, however, requires
careful monitoring and potential repeat doses to maintain the reversal
of the opioid effects. The interplay between pharmacodynamics and
pharmacokinetics is critical in determining treatment strategies.

The concept of drug interactions is another critical aspect of paramedic pharmacology. Drugs can interact with each other in various
ways, either enhancing or diminishing each other's effects. Additive effects occur when two drugs with similar actions produce a combined effect equal to the sum of their individual effects. Synergistic effects, on
the other hand, arise when the combined effect is greater than the sum
of individual effects. Antagonistic effects occur when one drug blocks
or reduces the effect of another. These interactions can have profound
consequences, sometimes leading to unexpected and potentially dangerous side effects.

A classic example is the interaction between benzodiazepines and
opioids. Both drug classes can cause respiratory depression, and their
combined use significantly increases the risk of respiratory failure. This
necessitates careful monitoring of respiratory rate and oxygen saturation when administering both medications. Similarly, the interaction
between certain antibiotics and anticoagulants can increase the risk of
bleeding. The thorough assessment of a patient's medication history is
therefore paramount, helping us anticipate and manage potential drug
interactions.

Moving beyond the theoretical, let's examine some commonly used medications in paramedic practice. Epinephrine, a potent sympathomimetic, is a cornerstone of managing anaphylaxis. Its ability to stimulate alpha-adrenergic receptors causes vasoconstriction, while its beta-adrenergic effects increase heart rate and bronchodilation, counteracting the life-threatening effects of anaphylaxis. Its administration must be meticulous, requiring precise dosing and close monitoring of the patient's vital signs. Improper administration can lead to serious cardiovascular consequences. Aspirin, an antiplatelet agent, plays a vital role in acute coronary syndromes, reducing platelet aggregation and improving blood flow to the heart. Again, careful consideration of potential bleeding risks is crucial.

Another example is adenosine, used to treat supraventricular tachycardia. Its rapid onset of action and short half-life necessitate intravenous administration, typically followed by a saline flush to ensure it reaches the heart quickly. Knowing the precise mechanisms of these drugs, as well as their limitations, allows us to make informed decisions about their use. Even seemingly straightforward medications like oxygen require a deep understanding. While oxygen is essential for life, administering it inappropriately, particularly to patients with certain lung conditions, can have unintended consequences. Similarly, the judicious use of analgesics, such as morphine or fentanyl, requires careful balancing of pain relief with the risk of respiratory depression. Our understanding of the physiological effects of pain and the potential for opioid-induced respiratory depression is crucial in providing safe and effective pain management.

Understanding contraindications is just as important as understanding indications. For example, beta-blockers are contraindicated in certain types of heart block, as they can exacerbate the condition. Knowing a patient's medical history and identifying potential contraindications is paramount before administering any medication. Moreover, the assessment of potential side effects is critical. Every medication carries a risk of side effects, some minor and others potentially life-threatening. Recognizing these potential side effects and being prepared to manage them is crucial for patient safety.

The administration of medications in the prehospital setting presents unique challenges. We often work in unpredictable environments with limited resources and under considerable time pressure. Maintaining sterile technique, correctly calculating dosages, and administering medications safely and effectively require a high level of skill and precision. Regular continuing education and the commitment to maintaining our clinical competencies are fundamental in ensuring our ability to provide safe and effective pharmacological interventions.

Furthermore, documentation of medication administration is crucial. Precise recording of the medication administered, the dose, the route of administration, the time of administration, and the patient's response is not just good practice, it is a legal requirement. Accurate and complete documentation provides a crucial record of our clinical interventions, essential for patient care continuity and legal protection.

In summary, pharmacology is a cornerstone of effective paramedic practice. It's a complex and evolving field requiring ongoing learning and a commitment to staying current with best practices. Our understanding extends beyond simple memorization; it encompasses a grasp of the underlying mechanisms of action, potential interactions, and potential adverse effects of the medications we administer. The emphasis on safe administration and meticulous documentation underscores the critical responsibility we bear in providing high-quality prehospital care. This comprehensive knowledge, combined with skillful application, empowers us to make life-saving interventions that significantly impact patient outcomes. The continual pursuit of knowledge and the application of critical thinking in the prehospital setting are critical factors in a paramedic's skillset, guaranteeing the delivery of high quality patient care.

Building on our understanding of pharmacology and its critical role in prehospital care, we now turn to a cornerstone of emergency medicine: Advanced Cardiac Life Support (ACLS). ACLS protocols represent the culmination of decades of research and clinical experience, offering a structured approach to managing the most critical cardiac emergencies. These protocols aren't rigid sets of rules, but rather frameworks designed to guide our decision-making in the chaotic and often unpredictable world of emergency response. They emphasize a systematic approach, combining rapid assessment, timely interventions, and continuous reassessment to maximize the chances of a successful outcome.

One of the most demanding scenarios we face is cardiac arrest. The sudden cessation of cardiac output, effectively halting the flow of oxygenated blood to vital organs, necessitates immediate and decisive action. The initial moments are critical; the longer the heart remains in standstill, the lower the chances of survival. ACLS protocols emphasize the importance of high-quality CPR, emphasizing proper chest compressions, adequate ventilation, and minimizing interruptions to maintain cerebral and myocardial perfusion.

Early defibrillation is paramount in many cases of cardiac arrest, particularly those involving ventricular fibrillation (VF) or pulseless ventricular tachycardia (pVT). These lethal rhythms need to be addressed promptly to restore a perfusing rhythm. The immediate deployment of an automated external defibrillator (AED) significantly improves survival rates, emphasizing the importance of public access defibrillation programs. Our role as paramedics extends beyond operating the AED;

we are responsible for ensuring its proper use, confirming the presence of shockable rhythms, and providing the necessary post-shock care.

Beyond defibrillation, effective ACLS relies heavily on a thorough understanding of cardiac pharmacology. Epinephrine, a potent sympathomimetic, plays a crucial role in many ACLS algorithms. It acts primarily on alpha-adrenergic receptors, causing vasoconstriction and improving coronary perfusion pressure. It also has beta-adrenergic effects, increasing heart rate and contractility. While essential, epinephrine's use requires careful consideration, as excessive doses can lead to detrimental cardiovascular effects such as increased myocardial oxygen demand and potentially fatal arrhythmias.

Another key medication in ACLS is amiodarone, an antiarrhythmic with a broader spectrum of action than epinephrine. It's effective in treating VF and pVT that are refractory to defibrillation and epinephrine. Amiodarone alters sodium and potassium channel activity, suppressing abnormal electrical activity in the heart. However, amiodarone carries potential side effects, including hypotension and bradycardia, necessitating careful monitoring. The administration of amiodarone must always be meticulously documented to ensure a clear record of the patient's treatment.

The importance of teamwork in ACLS cannot be overstated. Successful resuscitation often hinges on effective communication, clear roles, and coordinated action among the team members. Paramedics must be adept at leading and participating in a team environment, providing clear concise instructions, and effectively delegating tasks, all while maintaining situational awareness. I recall one particular incident where seamless teamwork was the difference between life and death. We responded to a call for a 60-year-old male found unresponsive in his home. Upon arrival, the patient was pulseless and apneic. The team, comprising myself, an EMT, and a firefighter, worked together seamlessly. While I initiated chest compressions and directed the EMT to attach the AED, the firefighter quickly established IV access. The rapid and coordinated actions enabled us to swiftly deliver the necessary interventions, eventually restoring a perfusing rhythm.

Beyond cardiac arrest, ACLS encompasses the management of other life-threatening cardiac conditions. For instance, unstable angina and acute myocardial infarction (AMI) demand rapid intervention to limit myocardial damage. The administration of nitroglycerin, a potent vasodilator, can help alleviate chest pain and improve myocardial perfusion. However, it's contraindicated in cases of hypotension or the potential for right ventricular infarct. Our understanding of the pathophysiology of these conditions is paramount in selecting appropriate interventions. We must assess vital signs, consider the patient's history, and interpret the electrocardiogram (ECG) to make informed decisions.

The effective management of acute coronary syndromes necessitates a seamless integration of prehospital and in-hospital care. In the prehospital setting, we focus on stabilizing the patient, minimizing further cardiac damage, and ensuring a rapid transfer to the appropriate facility. This involves initiating timely administration of medications, providing oxygen, monitoring vital signs, and providing emotional support to the patient and their family. Our actions in the prehospital setting directly impact the patient's prognosis and chances of long-term recovery.

Beyond the immediate management of cardiac emergencies, ACLS emphasizes the importance of post-resuscitation care. Patients who survive cardiac arrest often require ongoing support, including ventilation, medication management, and monitoring of vital signs. We must ensure that they are transported safely to a hospital equipped to provide specialized care, and we need to maintain close communication with the receiving hospital team to facilitate a smooth transition. Accurate and detailed documentation of all interventions, patient responses, and changes in vital signs is critical, providing the hospital team with a comprehensive overview of the situation and enhancing the continuity of care.

Furthermore, ACLS principles extend beyond the immediate resuscitation setting. We use principles of ACLS in the assessment and management of other critical conditions. For example, understanding the mechanisms of shock, whether hypovolemic, cardiogenic, or distributive, requires a strong foundation in ACLS concepts. Similarly, managing respiratory failure often involves aspects of ACLS, such as the administration of medications and the support of ventilation.

Reflecting on my own experiences, I can attest to the importance of continuing education and the continuous refinement of skills in ACLS. The field of cardiac care is constantly evolving, with new research and guidelines emerging regularly. Staying abreast of these advancements is crucial for maintaining high standards of care. We must continuously update our knowledge, participate in regular training programs, and embrace new technologies, such as improved defibrillators and monitoring equipment. One instance highlighted this: a new protocol for post-resuscitation care was implemented that significantly improved patient outcomes. The update involved a different administration regimen for certain medications and introduced new monitoring strategies. Embracing the change immediately improved our patient care.

In conclusion, Advanced Cardiac Life Support is not just a set of protocols but a dynamic and ever-evolving approach to managing life-threatening cardiac conditions. It requires a multifaceted approach, integrating a strong foundation in pharmacology, a systematic approach to patient assessment and management, excellent teamwork, and a commitment to continuous learning. Our ability to effectively manage these emergencies significantly influences patient outcomes, highlighting the importance of meticulous preparation, precise execution, and a commitment to excellence. This dedication to best practices and continuous improvement underscores the central role of ACLS in our daily practice, ensuring we provide the best possible care to patients in their most critical moments. The emotional and physical demands of this role necessitate self-care and a strong support network, reinforcing the need for personal well-being to sustain the intensity of this profession. The knowledge gained through experience, paired with an unwavering commitment to ongoing professional development, is what ultimately allows paramedics to navigate the complexities of ACLS and provide the best possible chance of survival for patients in cardiac arrest and other critical situations.

Trauma management represents a significant portion of a paramedic's workload, demanding a comprehensive understanding of the principles of trauma care. It's a realm where split-second decisions under immense pressure can dramatically impact a patient's outcome. Unlike the structured approach of ACLS, trauma management requires a more adaptable and holistic approach, prioritizing rapid assessment, immediate stabilization, and efficient transport to definitive care. The chaotic nature of a major trauma scene necessitates a systematic approach, often working in conjunction with other emergency services, underscoring the critical importance of teamwork and effective communication.

The initial assessment of a trauma patient is crucial, often dictated by the mechanism of injury (MOI). A high-energy impact, such as a motor vehicle collision at high speed, suggests a higher likelihood of significant internal injuries compared to a low-energy fall. This initial impression guides the priority of our interventions. We use the primary assessment, a rapid survey focused on identifying and addressing immediately life-threatening conditions. This includes checking for airway patency, breathing adequacy, and circulation, the ABCs that form the backbone of trauma care. Is the airway open and clear? Is the patient breathing effectively? Is there a palpable pulse, and if not, are effective compressions initiated immediately? Addressing these critical elements forms the foundation upon which all subsequent interventions are built.

Maintaining a patent airway is paramount. This may involve simple maneuvers like head tilt-chin lift or jaw thrust, or more advanced techniques such as endotracheal intubation or surgical cricothyroidotomy in cases of severe airway obstruction. The choice of technique depends on the patient's condition and the paramedic's skill set. I recall a scene involving a motorcyclist who suffered severe facial trauma. His airway was compromised, and we had to rapidly perform a rapid sequence intubation to secure his airway. The timely intervention undoubtedly saved his life. This highlights the importance of mastering advanced airway techniques and their rapid execution under duress.

Assessing breathing involves evaluating the rate, rhythm, depth, and effort of respiration. Inadequate breathing may require assisted ventilation with a bag-valve mask or advanced airway management. The use of supplemental oxygen is almost always indicated, aiming for a saturation above 94%. Auscultation of the lungs helps to identify the presence of breath sounds and detect any abnormalities such as wheezing, rhonchi, or absent sounds. These subtle indicators can pinpoint problems such as pneumothorax or hemothorax, both life-threatening conditions requiring prompt attention.

Evaluating circulation involves assessing pulse rate, quality, and blood pressure. A rapid, weak pulse might suggest hypovolemia (low blood volume) due to significant blood loss, while a low blood pressure indicates inadequate tissue perfusion. The presence of external bleeding requires immediate control to prevent further blood loss. Direct pressure, elevation, and tourniquets are the standard methods employed depending upon the nature and location of the bleeding. In massive haemorrhage, we often initiate large-bore intravenous access to administer fluids and blood products, if available. It's vital to remember that hypovolemic shock is a progressive condition, and early recognition and aggressive treatment are critical.

Once the primary assessment is complete, we proceed to the secondary assessment, a more detailed examination of the patient. This includes a systematic head-to-toe evaluation, searching for hidden injuries. While we prioritize life-threatening injuries first, recognizing the potential for injuries hidden beneath the surface is critical for effective trauma management. The secondary assessment might unveil injuries not readily apparent during the initial examination. For example, a patient with a seemingly minor fall might have sustained internal organ damage not visible externally.

In cases of multiple injuries, prioritizing treatment is essential. The use of the ATLS (Advanced Trauma Life Support) approach, a standardized protocol, is crucial in these scenarios. This involves a systematic approach to evaluating and managing trauma patients, ensuring that life-threatening injuries are addressed first. This organized approach is what separates effective trauma care from chaotic and potentially ineffective interventions. Applying ATLS principles allows us to methodically address issues, preventing overlooking potentially fatal problems during a stressful scene. Teamwork becomes paramount in these complex situations. Each team member must have a clear role and understanding of the overarching strategy.

During the secondary assessment, we obtain a detailed history from the patient or bystanders whenever possible. This includes the MOI, pre-existing medical conditions, and any allergies. This information adds context to the assessment and can help guide our management decisions. A thorough history, often gleaned from difficult circumstances, allows for better clinical judgement in tailoring treatment strategies.

The efficient transport of the trauma patient to the appropriate medical facility is a crucial component of trauma care. The selection of the destination hospital is often based on the patient's condition and the availability of specialized care. This decision is typically made in consultation with medical control, but the paramedic's assessment plays a critical role. For example, a patient with severe head injuries might require transport to a Level I trauma center, equipped to provide neurosurgical expertise. This collaboration with the medical control physician exemplifies teamwork in the field. Ensuring seamless transfer to the correct facility significantly impacts the patient's survival rates.

Communication is vital throughout the entire process. Clear and concise communication with the hospital, other emergency responders, and the patient's family is essential for a smooth and effective process. Providing timely updates and accurate information ensures a cohesive approach to care, minimizing delays and facilitating a seamless transition of care. This might involve relaying vital signs, interventions undertaken, and any significant changes in the patient's condition. Effective communication not only improves patient care, but also reduces stress for the entire team.

Beyond technical skills, effective trauma management requires empathy and compassion. Trauma patients often experience significant emotional distress, compounded by physical injuries. Providing emotional support and reassuring communication can significantly alleviate their suffering. This human element of paramedicine is often overlooked, yet it constitutes a vital part of comprehensive care. This empathetic approach is what separates a good paramedic from an outstanding one.

Finally, meticulous documentation is essential. Detailed records of the assessment, interventions, and patient's response are crucial for legal and medical reasons. This detailed documentation is also beneficial for further medical review, assisting in the development of best practices. It also serves as a crucial link in the chain of care, providing continuity of care between the pre-hospital and hospital settings. This aspect often goes beyond just factual reporting. It requires a thorough and systematic approach to recording observations and interventions.

Trauma management is a demanding but rewarding aspect of paramedicine. It demands a blend of technical skill, rapid decision-making, teamwork, and compassion. Continuous professional development and adherence to established protocols are vital for providing the highest quality of care to trauma patients. This continual learning and refinement of skills is essential for maintaining proficiency in this challenging area of prehospital care. The field of trauma care is continuously evolving, so staying up-to-date with the latest advances is paramount for providing the best possible patient care. This continuous dedication is what sets paramedics apart.

Respiratory emergencies form a significant and often terrifying aspect of paramedic practice. The sheer panic in a patient's eyes as they struggle for each breath, the audible wheeze or gasp, the desperate clinging to air – these images are etched into the memory of every paramedic. Managing these crises requires not only a deep understanding of respiratory physiology and pathophysiology, but also a calm, decisive approach that can quickly stabilize a deteriorating patient. Unlike the often-structured approach to trauma, respiratory emergencies can present with a bewildering array of symptoms and varying degrees of severity, demanding a flexible and adaptable response.

One of the most common respiratory emergencies we face is the asthma attack. The characteristic wheezing, shortness of breath, and cough are tell-tale signs, but the severity can range from mild to life-threatening. My first experience with a severe asthma attack was particularly impactful. A young woman, barely in her twenties, was found collapsed in her apartment, her face cyanotic, her breathing labored and whistling. Her inhaler lay discarded nearby, a testament to the escalating crisis she'd been unable to manage. That day, the speed and precision required to administer nebulized albuterol and administer supplemental oxygen felt like a frantic dance against time. We got her breathing under control, but the memory serves as a stark reminder of the critical nature of early intervention.

The initial assessment in asthma is crucial. We must evaluate the patient's level of distress, their respiratory rate and effort, their oxygen saturation levels, and the presence of any accessory muscle use. A patient struggling to breathe, using their intercostal and sternocleidomastoid muscles to aid inspiration, is clearly in significant respiratory distress. Auscultation of the lungs reveals the characteristic wheezing – the hallmark of bronchospasm. However, silent chest can also indicate severe airflow obstruction, a sign of impending respiratory failure requiring immediate intervention.

The cornerstone of asthma management is bronchodilation. Nebulized beta-agonists, such as albuterol, are our first line of defense, rapidly relaxing the smooth muscles in the bronchioles and opening up the airways. We administer this medication using a nebulizer, ensuring that the patient receives a consistent dose of the medication. The effect is usually quite rapid; within minutes, we should see an improvement in the patient's respiratory rate, effort, and oxygen saturation levels.

However, some patients may require more aggressive intervention. If the patient's condition does not improve with nebulized albuterol, we may consider adding ipratropium bromide, an anticholinergic medication that further dilates the airways. In severe cases, intravenous corticosteroids, such as methylprednisolone, can be administered to reduce inflammation in the airways, though their effects are not immediate. In rare instances, and only under the guidance of medical control, we might even consider administering magnesium sulfate, a bronchodilator and smooth muscle relaxant effective in refractory cases. The careful selection and administration of these medications are crucial, as any errors can have life-threatening consequences.

Beyond asthma, we encounter other respiratory emergencies, including pneumonia, which presents a different set of challenges. Pneumonia, an infection of the lungs typically involves a cough, fever, and shortness of breath. Unlike asthma, pneumonia may not present with classic wheezing; instead, you might hear crackles or rales during auscultation – the sounds of fluid in the alveoli. The patient's oxygen saturation levels may be significantly reduced, indicating hypoxemia, a life-threatening condition requiring immediate attention.

Our approach to pneumonia differs somewhat from managing asthma. While supplemental oxygen is crucial, we're primarily focused on supporting the patient's breathing and providing comfort measures until they can reach hospital care. We frequently employ non-invasive ventilation strategies, like a nasal cannula or high-flow oxygen therapy, depending on the patient's need. In certain scenarios, even non-rebreather masks may be necessary. While we can't cure pneumonia in the field, we can mitigate the effects of the disease and provide the best support until the patient reaches the appropriate level of care.

Another respiratory emergency that demands our immediate attention is acute respiratory distress syndrome (ARDS). This severe condition, often a consequence of severe trauma, sepsis, or other critical illnesses, involves widespread inflammation and fluid buildup in the lungs. ARDS patients present with extreme shortness of breath, rapid respiratory rates, low oxygen saturation levels, and often frothy sputum. They are critically ill and require immediate advanced care.

Managing ARDS pre-hospital is exceptionally challenging. Providing high-flow oxygen therapy and, in certain circumstances, non-invasive ventilation techniques is often the most we can do in the field. We also need to be hypervigilant to monitor the patient's oxygenation and respiratory status, constantly assessing for any deterioration. This demands a keen awareness and an unwavering focus on maintaining airway patency and providing appropriate respiratory support.

Beyond these specific conditions, there's a whole spectrum of respiratory emergencies, including pulmonary edema, pulmonary embolism, and even foreign body aspiration. Each of these requires a unique approach, demanding a deep understanding of pathophysiology and rapid decision-making. The common thread that ties them together is the need for prompt recognition, rapid intervention, and skillful management to preserve the patient's life. Often, our interventions are aimed not at curing the underlying condition, but at mitigating its effects and ensuring that the patient reaches definitive care as quickly and safely as possible.

Effective respiratory emergency management relies heavily on accurate and timely assessment. We must be adept at evaluating the patient's respiratory rate, rhythm, depth, and effort, auscultating their lungs, and monitoring their oxygen saturation levels. Any change in the patient's condition, however subtle, needs to be carefully evaluated and addressed appropriately. It's not uncommon to see a patient's condition deteriorate rapidly, underscoring the importance of continuous monitoring and vigilant observation.

Communication is another vital component. Clear and concise communication with the emergency department, medical control, and other emergency responders is crucial, ensuring a seamless transition of care. We must provide accurate and timely updates on the patient's condition, our interventions, and the patient's response, so the hospital can prepare for the patient's arrival and provide prompt, adequate care. Without effective communication, delays can occur, potentially endangering the patient's life.

Moreover, in respiratory emergencies, as in all aspects of paramedicine, detailed documentation is paramount. We must meticulously record our assessments, interventions, and the patient's response. These records are not merely administrative tasks; they serve as critical evidence, ensuring accountability, contributing to future learning and facilitating a thorough medical review. The meticulous details captured in our documentation serve as a link in the chain of care, ensuring consistent treatment and ultimately maximizing the chances of a positive outcome for the patient.

Finally, respiratory emergency management, like all areas of paramedicine, underscores the importance of continuous professional development. Regular training, staying abreast of the latest advances in medical knowledge and technology, and maintaining proficiency in advanced airway techniques are essential. It's a field that demands constant learning, refinement, and a commitment to excellence. The emotional toll of witnessing patients struggle for breath, coupled with the pressure of making critical decisions under duress, can be significant. Therefore, it's crucial to reflect on experiences, learn from mistakes, and develop a resilient mindset to handle the emotional and mental challenges inherent in this demanding profession. The reward, however, is immense – the satisfaction of saving a life and alleviating suffering, a powerful motivator in this demanding yet rewarding career.

12

The Business of Paramedicine

The adrenaline rush of a successful resuscitation, the quiet satisfaction of providing comfort to a grieving family, the camaraderie shared with colleagues during a long, exhausting shift – these are the moments that often define our perception of paramedicine. However, the reality of the profession extends far beyond the immediacy of the emergency response. It encompasses a complex web of legal and regulatory frameworks that govern our practice, protect our rights, and ensure the safety and well-being of both paramedics and the patients we serve. Understanding these frameworks is not just a matter of compliance; it's crucial for navigating the professional landscape, protecting ourselves from potential liabilities, and advocating for our own interests.

One of the most fundamental aspects of our professional lives is the employment contract. This seemingly straightforward document is actually a legally binding agreement that outlines the terms and conditions of our employment, including our responsibilities, salary, benefits, and working hours. It's a document that often gets overlooked, a contract quickly signed and filed away, only to be resurrected during moments of dispute or uncertainty. However, taking the time to meticulously read and understand every clause is crucial. A poorly understood or poorly drafted contract can lead to misunderstandings, disagreements, and even legal battles down the line.

I recall a colleague, early in his career, who signed a contract without carefully reviewing it. He later discovered a clause requiring mandatory overtime without adequate compensation. It wasn't until he experienced the relentless pressure of repeated mandatory overtime, impacting his personal life and mental well-being, that he realized the implications of his hasty decision. The subsequent legal battles proved lengthy, costly, and emotionally draining, highlighting the importance of due diligence in reviewing employment contracts.

Beyond the specifics of compensation and benefits, employment contracts often include critical details regarding working conditions, including provisions regarding safety equipment, training requirements, and disciplinary procedures. Understanding these clauses is vital for ensuring a safe and productive work environment. For example, the contract might outline the employer's responsibility for providing appropriate personal protective equipment (PPE), such as gloves, masks, and eye protection, to mitigate exposure to infectious diseases or hazardous materials. Similarly, it might detail the employer's commitment to providing ongoing professional development opportunities, crucial for maintaining competence and staying abreast of advancements in medical technology and procedures.

Moreover, employment contracts often address issues related to workplace conduct, including policies on harassment, discrimination, and professional ethics. These clauses help establish a respectful and professional work environment, safeguarding the interests of all employees. Understanding these policies is crucial not only for avoiding disciplinary action but also for fostering a culture of respect and accountability within the paramedic team. Knowing your rights and responsibilities is the foundation of a successful professional career.

Another critical area is worker's compensation, a system designed to protect employees injured on the job. This is an area where thorough understanding is paramount. Worker's compensation laws vary by jurisdiction, but they generally provide medical benefits and wage replacement for injuries sustained while performing job-related duties. The process of filing a worker's compensation claim can be complex, involving documentation, medical evaluations, and potentially legal representation. It is crucial to understand the specific requirements of your local worker's compensation board, and to meticulously document any injury or illness potentially related to your employment. Failure to do so can result in delays, denials of benefits, and further financial and emotional distress.

I remember one instance when a colleague suffered a back injury while lifting a patient. His initial claim was delayed due to inadequate documentation, leading to a significant gap in his income and prolonged recovery. This experience highlighted the importance of meticulous record-keeping, and prompted him to become an advocate for improved training and awareness among his peers regarding worker's compensation procedures. This situation emphasizes the need for proactive documentation and a thorough understanding of the legal framework to safeguard our well-being.

Union representation plays a vital role in protecting the rights and interests of paramedics. Unions negotiate collective bargaining agreements that define wages, benefits, working conditions, and other terms of employment. They also provide legal representation and support to members facing disciplinary action or grievances. In many jurisdictions, unions are instrumental in advocating for improvements in workplace safety, working conditions, and employee benefits. The collective power of a union can provide a crucial safeguard against exploitation and ensure fair treatment for all members.

In some cases, paramedics may be faced with ethical dilemmas that bring them into conflict with their employers or other entities. For instance, there might be situations where paramedics are pressured to compromise their clinical judgment or violate ethical guidelines. Understanding the relevant legal and regulatory frameworks, including whistleblower protection laws, is essential for navigating such complex situations. These laws are designed to protect healthcare professionals who report unethical or illegal activities within their workplace. However, these processes can also be complicated and require careful planning and execution. Seeking legal advice from a professional specializing in healthcare law is always prudent in such complex situations. The protection these laws offer is not automatic; it requires a clear understanding of one's rights and responsibilities.

Beyond employment contracts and unions, paramedics must be aware of other relevant regulations, including those related to patient confidentiality (HIPAA in the US), data privacy, and the use of emergency medical equipment. Violations of these regulations can have severe consequences, including fines, disciplinary action, and even criminal charges. Continuous professional development should incorporate regular review of these regulations to ensure compliance and maintain a high standard of ethical conduct. The field of paramedicine is constantly evolving, with new technologies, procedures, and regulations emerging regularly. Staying informed and updated is a crucial aspect of our professional responsibilities.

Furthermore, the legal landscape surrounding paramedicine is dynamic and constantly evolving. State and federal laws, as well as court decisions, can significantly impact our professional practice. It's therefore crucial to stay informed about any changes or updates to these regulations. Professional organizations and legal resources can provide valuable information and support in navigating this evolving legal landscape. Seeking guidance from legal professionals experienced in healthcare law provides valuable support and can help prevent potential misunderstandings or costly errors.

In conclusion, while the thrill and immediate gratification of saving lives forms the core of our work, a robust understanding of employment contracts, regulations, and legal protections is equally crucial. It is an integral part of our professional responsibilities and contributes to the security and sustainability of our careers. This knowledge not only safeguards our own interests but also ensures we can continue to provide the highest quality of care, free from undue pressure or risk. Investing time and effort in understanding this multifaceted area isn't simply about avoiding trouble; it's about empowering ourselves to navigate the complexities of the profession, advocating for our rights, and ultimately, providing the best possible care for our patients. The combination of clinical skills, compassionate care, and a clear understanding of the legal and ethical frameworks allows paramedics to excel in our roles. It's not just about knowing how to treat a patient, but also how to protect ourselves and uphold the integrity of the profession.

Negotiating salaries and benefits is often a daunting prospect, especially for those entering the field or lacking experience in such discussions. However, understanding your worth and advocating for fair compensation is a crucial skill for any paramedic. It's not simply about the numbers on a paycheck; it's about recognizing the value you bring to the system and ensuring a sustainable, healthy career. Many paramedics, particularly those early in their careers, feel uncomfortable negotiating. We're often trained to prioritize patient care above all else, sometimes at the expense of our own needs. This selflessness, while admirable, can leave us vulnerable to undercompensation and unfair working conditions. Remember, your well-being is as important as the well-being of your patients. Burnout is a real and pervasive threat in our profession, and adequate compensation and benefits are essential for mitigating its effects.

One of the first steps involves thorough research. Understanding the salary ranges for paramedics in your region and with similar experience is crucial. Websites like Salary.com, Glassdoor, and Indeed can offer valuable insights. Furthermore, speaking with colleagues, networking with others in the field, and checking union websites (if applicable) can provide a more nuanced picture of local compensation trends. This research allows you to enter a negotiation with informed confidence, knowing your worth and the market value of your skills. Don't just focus on the base salary. Consider the entire benefits package, including health insurance, retirement contributions, paid time off, and continuing education opportunities. These perks can significantly impact your overall financial well-being and professional development.

When preparing for a salary negotiation, it's helpful to quantify your accomplishments. Create a list highlighting your skills, certifications, and experience. Did you successfully complete advanced training? Do you have a specialized skill set like critical care transport or wilderness medicine? Have you consistently received positive performance reviews? Quantify your successes whenever possible. Instead of simply stating "I'm a highly skilled paramedic," articulate it as "In my three years of experience, I've successfully managed over 500 critical calls, resulting in consistently positive patient outcomes." These concrete examples provide compelling evidence of your value.

The negotiation itself should be a professional and respectful conversation. Start by expressing your interest in the position and reiterating your enthusiasm for the opportunity. Then, clearly and confidently state your desired salary range, based on your research and accomplishments. This is not a time for timidity. Present your case with the data you've collected, showing you understand the market value of your skills. Be prepared to discuss your contributions and justify your requested compensation. If the initial offer is lower than your desired range, don't be afraid to counter with a reasoned proposal. Highlight the unique skills and value you bring to the organization. Consider suggesting a compromise, but only if it aligns with your minimum requirements. For instance, you might be willing to accept a slightly lower salary in exchange for additional paid time off or enhanced benefits.

Remember, negotiation is a two-way street. The employer is also considering their budget and the value they perceive you bring. Finding common ground is often the key to a successful outcome.

It's also important to consider the long-term implications of your salary and benefits package. Think beyond the immediate financial gain. Consider the impact of employer-sponsored retirement plans and health insurance on your long-term financial security. A comprehensive benefits package can provide crucial peace of mind, reducing stress and financial strain in the future. This is especially crucial in a profession known for its high stress levels and potential for burnout. Consider aspects like disability insurance, which is essential given the physical demands of the job. Protecting your health and your financial future is not a luxury; it is a necessity.

Many paramedics benefit from union representation. Unions negotiate collective bargaining agreements that establish minimum salary standards, benefits packages, and working conditions. They also provide legal assistance and advocate for improved workplace safety and fairer employment practices. If your employer is unionized, becoming a member provides a powerful voice in advocating for your rights and interests. The collective power of a union can significantly improve your bargaining position and ensure fair treatment for all members. Even in non-unionized workplaces, forming a network of colleagues can provide collective bargaining power. Sharing information about salary and benefits, and discussing concerns collectively can create a powerful force for change. This collaborative approach can be particularly effective in addressing systemic issues, such as inadequate staffing levels or unsafe working conditions.

One aspect often overlooked is the importance of continuous professional development. Invest in your skills and knowledge. Advanced certifications, specialized training, and continuing education not only enhance your job performance but also increase your marketability. This can be used as leverage during salary negotiations. Highlighting your commitment to ongoing learning demonstrates your dedication to the profession and your desire to provide the best possible care. The return on investment in your professional development is significant, not just in terms of salary, but also in job satisfaction and career advancement. Employers value employees who demonstrate a commitment to lifelong learning and professional growth.

Beyond financial compensation, consider the overall work-life balance offered by a potential employer. High stress levels, long shifts, and exposure to traumatic events are intrinsic to the job. Therefore, factors such as adequate paid time off, scheduling flexibility, and access to mental health resources become essential considerations when evaluating a job offer. A supportive work environment that prioritizes well-being is invaluable for mitigating burnout and maintaining a healthy work-life balance. It's a crucial factor to negotiate for, as it impacts not only your immediate well-being but also your long-term career sustainability.

Sometimes, you may need to consider leaving your current employer for better opportunities. Job searching should be a proactive process, not something done only when desperate. Network with other paramedics, attend conferences, and keep an eye on job postings. Having options allows you to leverage opportunities to gain better compensation and work conditions. Prepare a professional resume and cover letter that showcases your skills and accomplishments. Practice your interview skills, focusing on highlighting your value and demonstrating your knowledge of the market rates for your skills.

Finally, remember that advocating for yourself is not selfish. It's a professional necessity. Paramedics work in high-pressure, often dangerous, environments, facing both physical and emotional challenges. Fair compensation reflects the risks we take, the skills we possess, and the dedication we exhibit daily. Don't undervalue yourself; you deserve fair treatment and appropriate compensation for the vital work you do. Negotiating your salary and benefits isn't just about the money; it's about ensuring a sustainable and rewarding career in a demanding profession, allowing you to not only continue providing exceptional patient care, but also to prioritize your own well-being, allowing for longevity and preventing burnout.

The demanding nature of paramedicine extends beyond the physical and emotional toll; it significantly impacts our financial well-being. Unlike many professions with predictable schedules and consistent income, our work often involves irregular hours, on-call shifts, and the potential for overtime, making financial planning a complex but crucial element of a successful career. Ignoring this aspect can lead to chronic stress, hindering our ability to provide optimal patient care and jeopardizing our long-term financial security. This section will delve into practical strategies for managing finances within the unique context of paramedic work.

One of the first steps towards sound financial management is creating a realistic budget. This isn't about restrictive deprivation; it's about understanding where your money goes and making informed choices. Start by meticulously tracking your income and expenses for a few months. Use budgeting apps, spreadsheets, or even a simple notebook to record every transaction. Be honest with yourself; it's easy to overlook small expenses that can add up significantly over time. Once you have a clear picture of your spending habits, you can identify areas where you can cut back.

Many paramedics find that irregular work schedules make budgeting more challenging. One effective strategy is to budget based on your average monthly income rather than your fluctuating weekly income. This provides a more stable baseline for planning your expenses. You can also create a "cushion" or emergency fund to cover unexpected fluctuations in income or expenses. This buffer will help you avoid relying on high-interest credit cards or loans to cover unexpected costs.

Beyond budgeting, saving is paramount. Ideally, you should aim to save a portion of each paycheck, even if it seems small at first. Start by setting a realistic savings goal, such as saving a certain percentage of your income each month. Many financial experts recommend aiming for at least 20%, but even a smaller percentage is a significant start. Automate your savings by setting up automatic transfers from your checking account to your savings account. This makes saving effortless and ensures consistency.

Consider opening a high-yield savings account to maximize the returns on your savings. While interest rates may not be exceptionally high, it's better than letting your money sit idle in a regular checking account. Explore different banking options to find the best interest rates and features for your needs. Remember, the power of compound interest is significant over the long term. The earlier you start saving and investing, the greater the potential for growth.

Investing can seem intimidating, but it is a crucial aspect of long-term financial security. While the stock market can be volatile, investing allows your money to potentially grow faster than inflation, preserving its purchasing power over time. Many paramedics initially shy away from investing due to the complexity or fear of risk. Start by educating yourself about different investment options, such as index funds, mutual funds, or individual stocks. Consider working with a financial advisor who can help you create a diversified portfolio that aligns with your risk tolerance and financial goals.

Diversification is key to mitigating risk in investing. Don't put all your eggs in one basket. Spread your investments across different asset classes to minimize the impact of potential losses in any single investment. A mix of stocks, bonds, and real estate can provide a balanced approach. Many employers offer retirement plans, such as 401(k)s or 403(b)s, with matching contributions. These plans offer significant tax advantages and can significantly enhance your retirement savings. Always take advantage of employer matching contributions; it's essentially free money.

Debt management is another crucial area of financial planning for paramedics. High-interest debt, such as credit card debt, can quickly spiral out of control. Create a plan to pay down high-interest debt as quickly as possible. Consider strategies like the debt snowball or debt avalanche methods, depending on your preferences and financial situation. The debt snowball method focuses on paying off the smallest debts first for psychological motivation, while the debt avalanche method prioritizes paying off the highest-interest debts first to save money on interest payments.

Beyond personal debt, managing student loan debt is a significant concern for many paramedics. Explore different repayment options, such as income-driven repayment plans, which adjust your monthly payments based on your income. Consolidation options can simplify your payments and potentially lower your overall interest rate. Understanding your rights and options regarding student loan repayment is crucial.

Protecting yourself against unexpected expenses and life events is essential. Health insurance is a necessity, particularly in a profession with inherent physical risks. Consider supplemental health insurance options to cover gaps in your primary coverage. Disability insurance is equally vital, protecting your income if you become unable to work due to injury or illness. Life insurance provides financial security for your loved ones in case of your untimely death. Review your insurance coverage regularly to ensure it aligns with your needs and financial circumstances.

Tax planning is also a critical component of financial management. As paramedics, we have specific tax deductions and credits available to us. Consult with a tax professional to maximize your tax benefits and minimize your tax liability. They can help you understand tax deductions related to medical expenses, continuing education, and other professional expenses. Staying informed about changes in tax laws is also crucial to ensure you are taking advantage of all available deductions and credits.

Estate planning is often overlooked, but it's crucial for securing your family's financial future. Having a will ensures your assets are distributed according to your wishes. Consider other estate planning tools, such as trusts, to protect your assets and minimize estate taxes. Consulting with an estate planning attorney is advisable to ensure your plans are legally sound and effectively protect your family's interests.

Finally, remember that financial planning is an ongoing process. Regularly review your budget, savings goals, and investment strategy. Adjust your plans as your circumstances change. Attend workshops, read financial literature, or seek professional guidance to stay informed and make sound financial decisions. Financial stability is not a destination; it is a journey.

Remember, financial security is not simply about accumulating wealth; it's about creating a sense of control over your financial future, allowing you to navigate life's challenges and opportunities with confidence. This, in turn, improves your overall well-being, enabling you to better handle the physical and emotional demands of paramedicine and fostering resilience and job satisfaction. It's an investment in your professional longevity and your overall happiness. By proactively managing your finances, you invest not only in your future but also in your ability to continue providing exceptional patient care.

The financial groundwork laid in the previous section—budgeting, saving, investing, and debt management—forms a critical foundation for long-term career success in paramedicine. Financial stability provides the security needed to pursue opportunities for professional growth and advancement, minimizing the stress associated with career decisions. It's a critical element of our professional well-being, allowing us to focus on the job itself and not be constantly preoccupied with financial worries. This is especially pertinent in a field where long hours, unpredictable schedules, and potential for emotional toll often impact an individual's ability to dedicate themselves fully to furthering their career trajectory.

Career advancement in paramedicine isn't just about climbing the ladder; it's about expanding skills, deepening expertise, and increasing our contribution to the field. It's about finding fulfillment in the work we do and recognizing the long-term implications of our career choices. Many paramedics start with a strong sense of purpose, wanting to help people in their most vulnerable moments. This initial idealism, however, can be challenged by the realities of the job—the constant exposure to trauma, the demanding shifts, and the emotional weight of the experiences we witness. While maintaining that initial idealism is critical, so too is recognizing the need for personal and professional growth. This will enable sustained passion and job satisfaction.

One pathway to career advancement is through specialized training. Consider certifications in areas like critical care transport, flight paramedicine, or tactical emergency medical services (TEMS). These certifications demonstrate a commitment to excellence and open doors to higher-paying positions and increased responsibility. Remember, the investment in specialized training, while requiring financial resources, is an investment in your long-term career prospects. I recall a colleague, Sarah, who initially felt apprehensive about the financial commitment of becoming a flight paramedic. However, after careful budgeting and leveraging some of her savings, she pursued the certification and quickly saw a return on her investment, not just financially, but in the profound fulfillment she derived from her new role.

Beyond specialized certifications, paramedics can pursue leadership roles within their organizations. This might involve becoming a field training officer (FTO), mentoring new recruits, or taking on responsibilities in quality assurance or quality improvement programs. These positions are not only more lucrative but also provide an opportunity to impact the overall effectiveness of your EMS agency. Leading a team requires different skillsets, emphasizing communication, problem-solving, and conflict resolution, aspects often overlooked in the day-to-day demands of patient care. Furthermore, these leadership opportunities allow us to hone our soft skills, crucial for effective collaboration and teamwork.

Many paramedics are finding fulfilling opportunities in management positions within EMS agencies, private ambulance services, or hospital systems. This path requires a strategic approach, combining operational experience with business acumen. Mastering the managerial aspects of paramedicine, understanding budgetary constraints, scheduling, and personnel management are all necessary components of this progression. A good manager can improve not only the efficiency of an ambulance service but also the quality of patient care and the overall well-being of the team. The financial benefits are usually substantial, but just as importantly, a capable manager can help build a more supportive, positive, and less stressful work environment.

Another avenue for career advancement is moving into roles beyond the direct provision of patient care. This could include roles in medical administration, healthcare consulting, medical sales, or even pursuing a career in health policy and advocacy. Many paramedics' unique perspective and experience are highly valued in these arenas. The transition might involve further education, possibly a Master's degree in public health, health administration, or a related field. This demonstrates a commitment to ongoing professional development, essential for career mobility. These non-clinical roles can be equally, if not more, rewarding and can offer financial stability and significant job satisfaction.

Networking is an often underestimated but crucial aspect of career advancement. Building relationships with colleagues, supervisors, and mentors can open doors to new opportunities. Attending conferences, joining professional organizations like the National Association of Emergency Medical Technicians (NAEMT) or the National Association of State EMS Officials (NASEMSO), and participating in industry events can expand your network and keep you abreast of current trends and opportunities. Such engagement keeps your professional knowledge current and builds valuable relationships that can lead to unexpected career openings.

Moreover, continuing education is paramount. Paramedicine is a dynamic field, constantly evolving with advancements in medical technology and treatment protocols. Staying current with the latest research and techniques not only benefits your patients but also enhances your professional value. Taking advantage of continuing education opportunities, whether through online courses, workshops, or advanced certifications, demonstrates a commitment to lifelong learning and professional growth. This ongoing investment in your education enhances your marketability and opens up more professional possibilities. It shows a dedication that employers value highly.

It's crucial to remember that career advancement is not a linear path. There will be setbacks and unexpected turns. It's important to view these as learning opportunities and adjust your strategies accordingly. Resilience and adaptability are key qualities for any paramedic, in the field and in their professional growth trajectory. The skills and experience you accumulate over your career are invaluable assets. Do not be afraid to explore different paths and embrace challenges as opportunities for personal and professional development.

While financial security is an essential element in pursuing career advancement, it's also crucial to prioritize your well-being. The demanding nature of paramedicine takes a toll, both physically and emotionally. Burnout is a real threat. It's imperative to maintain a healthy work-life balance, prioritize self-care, and seek support when needed. This is not a sign of weakness; rather, it's a testament to a commitment to longevity in the profession. A sustainable career requires that we attend to our own mental and physical health. It's impossible to excel professionally without prioritising personal well-being.

Finally, remember that your career journey is unique. What might work for one paramedic might not work for another. Consider your personal values, aspirations, and strengths when planning your career trajectory. Set realistic goals, break them down into smaller, achievable steps, and celebrate your milestones along the way. Regularly review and reassess your career plan, allowing for flexibility and adaptation. The field of paramedicine offers a myriad of career paths, and the key is to find the path that best aligns with your individual goals and aspirations. With thoughtful planning, a commitment to continuing education, and a focus on self-care, you can achieve both professional success and personal fulfillment. The journey might not always be easy, but the rewards of contributing to the community and making a real difference are immeasurable.

The traditional career path for a paramedic often involves climbing the ranks within a large EMS agency, progressing from EMT to paramedic, perhaps specializing in critical care or flight medicine. However, the landscape of emergency medical services is evolving, and increasingly, paramedics are finding fulfilling and financially rewarding careers by venturing into entrepreneurship. This presents a fascinating alternative to the traditional employment model, allowing for greater control over one's career trajectory and the potential for significantly higher earning potential.

One increasingly popular entrepreneurial path is establishing a private ambulance service. This requires a significant investment of time, capital, and meticulous planning, but the rewards can be substantial. First and foremost is the development of a robust business plan. This isn't simply a matter of purchasing ambulances and hiring staff; it necessitates a deep understanding of market analysis, identifying underserved areas or niches within the EMS market. For example, specialized transport services for high-acuity patients requiring advanced life support, or perhaps catering to a specific demographic like the elderly or those with complex medical needs, could prove highly lucrative. This requires thorough market research, identifying the specific needs of the community and developing a service to meet those needs effectively and efficiently. This research might involve studying demographics, analyzing competitor services, and assessing the regulatory landscape – licenses, permits and insurance requirements vary considerably between jurisdictions.

Securing funding is another critical hurdle. This could involve seeking loans from banks, securing investment from venture capitalists, or exploring government grants specifically designated for healthcare initiatives. Developing a convincing business plan that highlights the service's unique value proposition, demonstrates market viability, and projects a realistic financial return on investment is crucial in attracting investors. I remember a colleague, Mark, who successfully launched a private ambulance service specializing in non-emergency medical transportation. He painstakingly researched the local market, identified a gap in services for elderly patients requiring regular transport to dialysis appointments, and crafted a business plan that showcased this niche and the potential for substantial recurring revenue. His meticulous planning, coupled with his passion for patient care, secured him the necessary funding.

Beyond securing funding, the operational aspects of running a private ambulance service demand significant attention to detail. This includes the procurement and maintenance of ambulances, adhering to stringent safety and regulatory requirements, recruiting and retaining qualified personnel, managing payroll and insurance costs, and ensuring efficient scheduling and dispatch systems. Effective communication and management are vital in coordinating the various facets of the business. Moreover, building strong relationships with hospitals, nursing homes, and other healthcare providers is essential to secure patient referrals and maintain a steady flow of work. This requires both a skilled business acumen and the ability to build and cultivate networks within the healthcare community.

Another entrepreneurial avenue for paramedics is consulting. The unique expertise and experience gained in the field are highly valuable to various organizations within the healthcare sector. Consulting can encompass a wide range of services: advising on emergency preparedness for businesses or large events, providing expert witness testimony in legal cases involving medical negligence, offering training and educational programs for other EMS agencies, or conducting quality improvement audits for hospital emergency departments. Paramedics' practical, real-world experience is often in high demand for consulting engagements.

To establish a successful consulting business, a strong professional network is essential. This involves actively participating in industry conferences, engaging with professional organizations, and building rapport with potential clients. A well-crafted website or online portfolio showcasing one's expertise and experience is a crucial tool for marketing services. Furthermore, obtaining relevant certifications or advanced training, such as a Master's degree in public health or healthcare administration, can significantly enhance credibility and marketability. I've seen several colleagues successfully transition into consulting roles, leveraging their skills and knowledge to provide valuable services to hospitals, insurance companies, and even law enforcement agencies.

Beyond private ambulance services and consulting, paramedics can explore other entrepreneurial ventures within the EMS field. This might include developing and marketing specialized medical equipment, creating online educational resources for paramedics and EMTs, or designing mobile applications aimed at improving patient care or streamlining administrative processes. The key is identifying a need within the EMS sector and developing innovative solutions to meet that need. This entrepreneurial spirit, combined with a deep understanding of the EMS field, can lead to highly rewarding and fulfilling careers.

The path of entrepreneurship is not without its challenges. The initial investment required, both in time and finances, can be significant. The risk of financial failure is a factor that needs to be carefully considered. Moreover, managing the various aspects of a business – from financial planning and marketing to human resources and regulatory compliance – demands a diverse skillset and a high level of dedication. It's crucial to acknowledge the potential for setbacks and to develop a robust contingency plan to mitigate risk.

However, the potential rewards are substantial. Entrepreneurship offers the autonomy to design a career that aligns with personal values and aspirations. It provides the opportunity to build something from the ground up, fostering a deep sense of accomplishment and ownership. The financial rewards can also be significantly higher than traditional employment models within EMS.

Ultimately, the decision to pursue an entrepreneurial path within EMS requires careful self-reflection. It demands assessing one's skills, resources, and risk tolerance. A thorough business plan, meticulous market research, and a resilient mindset are crucial for success. However, for those willing to embrace the challenges, entrepreneurship in the EMS sector presents a dynamic and potentially highly rewarding alternative career path, demonstrating the ever-evolving possibilities for paramedics beyond the traditional roles. The ability to combine practical field experience with business acumen opens up a world of opportunity, a world where paramedics aren't just providers of emergency care, but also innovators and entrepreneurs shaping the future of the EMS profession. This transformation is a testament to the adaptability and entrepreneurial spirit within the EMS community, continually seeking new ways to serve the public and to find professional fulfillment. The paramedics I've known who've taken this leap have often found a level of job satisfaction and fulfillment that surpasses their expectations, a testament to the potential that lies in entrepreneurial endeavors within this demanding yet rewarding field.

13

Staying Current: Continuing Education

The adrenaline rush, the immediate life-or-death decisions, the camaraderie – these are the aspects of paramedicine that often draw individuals to the profession. But the reality extends far beyond the initial excitement. The constant evolution of medical knowledge, the emergence of new technologies, and the ever-shifting landscape of emergency medical services (EMS) demand a commitment to lifelong learning. This commitment manifests itself most concretely in the pursuit of Continuing Education Units (CEUs). CEUs aren't merely a box to tick; they represent a crucial investment in professional competence, patient safety, and personal growth. Neglecting them is akin to neglecting the very foundation upon which our practice rests.

My own journey highlights this. Early in my career, I approached CEUs with a certain level of apathy. They felt like an extra burden, an added administrative task tacked onto an already demanding schedule. I'd often cram for the required courses just before the renewal deadline, skimming through the materials rather than engaging deeply with the content. This superficial approach, I soon realized, was a disservice to both myself and my patients. A pivotal moment came during a particularly complex cardiac arrest. My instincts were sound, my training was adequate, but a subtle shift in treatment protocols, a nuance I'd missed in my rushed CEU review, could have potentially improved the outcome. That incident served as a brutal wake-up call. From then on, I approached continuing education with a far greater sense of responsibility and appreciation. I actively sought out challenging courses, delved into the research behind updated protocols, and fostered a culture of lifelong learning amongst my colleagues.

The benefits of active participation in continuing education are manifold and extend beyond mere compliance with licensing requirements. First and foremost, it ensures that we remain at the forefront of medical advances. The field of emergency medicine is dynamic, with constant advancements in pharmacology, diagnostic techniques, and treatment protocols. Ignoring these advancements is not only unprofessional but potentially dangerous. Regular engagement with CEUs allows us to integrate these new developments seamlessly into our practice, enhancing our ability to provide the highest level of care to patients in need. This continuous learning keeps us sharp, adaptable, and prepared for any situation we might encounter.

Furthermore, CEUs offer opportunities to specialize in specific areas of interest. Perhaps you find a particular fascination with pediatrics, toxicology, or trauma care. CEUs allow you to delve deeper into these areas, expanding your knowledge base and refining your skills. This specialization not only enhances your proficiency in your chosen area but also broadens your career prospects. I've seen colleagues, initially drawn to general paramedicine, discover a passion for critical care transport or wilderness medicine through specialized CEU courses, leading them to fulfilling and highly skilled roles.

The options for earning CEUs are surprisingly diverse, reflecting the multifaceted nature of the paramedic profession. Traditional classroom settings remain a valuable option, providing structured learning and the opportunity for direct interaction with instructors and peers. However, the availability of online courses has revolutionized the accessibility of continuing education. These courses offer flexibility, allowing paramedics to learn at their own pace and schedule, perfectly suited to the often irregular hours of paramedic work. I've found many on-line courses to be exceptionally well-designed and engaging, incorporating interactive simulations, video lectures, and case studies to provide a comprehensive learning experience. This flexibility is a game changer, especially for paramedics with families or other commitments that restrict their availability for traditional classroom instruction.

Conferences and workshops represent another significant avenue for CEU acquisition. These events provide valuable networking opportunities, allowing paramedics to connect with colleagues, industry experts, and researchers. The opportunity to engage in discussions, share experiences, and learn from the expertise of others is invaluable. Attending conferences also exposes paramedics to cutting-edge research and emerging trends, often before these insights find their way into mainstream textbooks or online courses. I recall one conference where I learned about a groundbreaking new technique for managing pediatric airway emergencies, a technique that I've since successfully implemented several times in the field. The immediate applicability of this knowledge significantly impacted my patient care capabilities.

Beyond formal educational settings, many opportunities exist for informal continuing education. This includes actively engaging in peer review, participating in quality improvement initiatives, and self-directed learning. Peer review, particularly with seasoned colleagues, provides valuable feedback and perspectives, helping us identify areas for improvement in our practice. Participating in quality improvement projects allows us to contribute to improvements within our own EMS systems, leading to enhanced efficiency and patient outcomes. Self-directed learning, such as reading professional journals, engaging in online forums, and researching specific clinical cases, keeps us abreast of the latest research and developments, further enriching our knowledge and skills. These less formal avenues are equally, if not more, valuable than traditional courses, particularly since they encourage a culture of ongoing self-reflection and continuous professional development.

The importance of CEUs extends beyond the purely technical aspects of paramedicine. They also offer opportunities to enhance leadership skills, communication skills, and stress management techniques. Effective communication is critical in interacting with patients, families, and other healthcare providers, and CEUs specifically focused on this skill can vastly improve patient outcomes. Similarly, courses on stress management and resilience build essential coping mechanisms, safeguarding the mental health and well-being of paramedics, a critical component in the face of the demanding and emotionally challenging aspects of the job. Neglecting these crucial aspects of continuing education leaves paramedics susceptible to burnout and compromises their overall effectiveness.

In conclusion, continuing education units are not simply a regulatory requirement; they are the lifeblood of a thriving paramedic career. They represent a commitment to continuous learning, professional growth, and ultimately, superior patient care.

Embracing the diverse opportunities for CEUs—from online courses and conferences to self-directed learning and peer review—is essential for remaining at the cutting edge of medical practice and ensuring the safety and well-being of both paramedics and the patients they serve. The investment of time and effort in acquiring CEUs is an investment in ourselves, our profession, and the future of emergency medical services. It's a commitment I wholeheartedly recommend – a commitment I've found has not only enhanced my professional abilities but also enriched my personal satisfaction in a career that consistently demands our very best. The journey of continuous learning, while demanding, is ultimately rewarding and essential for remaining a competent, compassionate, and confident paramedic in today's ever-evolving healthcare landscape.

The rapid pace of advancement in medicine presents a unique challenge and opportunity for paramedics. Staying abreast of the latest research, treatment protocols, and technological innovations is not merely a professional obligation; it's a critical component of providing optimal patient care and ensuring personal professional growth. The consequences of failing to keep current can be severe, ranging from suboptimal treatment outcomes to potentially life-threatening errors. I've witnessed firsthand the impact of outdated knowledge on patient care, a stark reminder of the imperative to engage in continuous learning.

One incident stands out vividly in my memory. We responded to a call for a young woman experiencing a severe allergic reaction. My initial assessment revealed classic symptoms: anaphylaxis. However, I relied on a protocol I'd learned several years prior, focusing on the administration of epinephrine and monitoring vital signs. While this approach was standard practice at the time, recent research had highlighted the potential benefits of using additional adjunctive therapies, such as high-flow oxygen and intravenous fluids. Had I been aware of these updated protocols, I could have potentially provided more comprehensive and effective treatment. While the patient ultimately recovered, the experience underscored the critical need for continuous learning and adaptation.

The methods for staying up-to-date are diverse and multifaceted, extending far beyond the traditional CEU courses. While CEUs remain a cornerstone of maintaining licensure and professional competency, they are just one piece of the larger puzzle. Active participation in professional organizations provides invaluable access to the latest research and ongoing discussions within the field. Membership in organizations like the National Association of Emergency Medical Technicians (NAEMT) or your local EMS association provides opportunities to network with colleagues, attend conferences, and receive regular updates on critical advancements. These organizations often publish newsletters, journals, and online resources specifically designed to keep members informed about significant changes in practice.

Journal articles form a significant component of staying informed. High-impact journals like the *Annals of Emergency Medicine* and *Prehospital Emergency Care* regularly publish research findings and clinical guidelines that directly impact prehospital care. However, simply reading abstracts is insufficient; critically reviewing the methodology, results, and conclusions is essential for proper integration into practice. This deeper level of engagement requires a commitment to scholarly inquiry and thoughtful reflection. It's a commitment that necessitates a significant time investment, yet its rewards are far-reaching.

Online resources have revolutionized the accessibility of medical information. Websites of reputable organizations such as the American Heart Association (AHA), American College of Cardiology (ACC), and various other specialized medical bodies provide readily available guidelines, updated protocols, and continuing education materials. Many of these resources offer free access to guidelines, summaries, and educational materials, making them indispensable tools for staying current. However, caution must be exercised, carefully vetting sources to ensure credibility and accuracy. The internet's abundance of information also includes misinformation, so discerning credible sources from unreliable ones is a vital skill. I've found it beneficial to stick to established, peer-reviewed sources, and cross-referencing information across multiple sources ensures a more complete and balanced understanding.

Conferences and workshops, as previously mentioned, offer a unique blend of formal and informal learning. These events provide opportunities to network with experts, hear presentations on cutting-edge research, and learn from the experiences of seasoned colleagues. The collaborative nature of these gatherings fosters a sense of community and allows for the exchange of best practices. I've frequently found myself learning as much from informal conversations and networking sessions as from the scheduled presentations. These conferences often serve as a platform for unveiling new technologies and techniques, offering a glimpse into the future of paramedicine.

Furthermore, participating in quality improvement initiatives within your own EMS system provides valuable insights into local trends and challenges. By actively contributing to these projects, paramedics can identify areas for improvement, participate in evidence-based practice, and refine existing protocols to reflect local needs. These initiatives provide a direct link between research and clinical practice, reinforcing the importance of continuous learning and adaptation.

Beyond formal channels, self-directed learning plays a crucial role. This includes reading professional journals, conducting online research, and actively seeking out cases and studies relevant to your practice area. Regular review of your own case notes and a self-reflective analysis of your performance can reveal areas for improvement and opportunities for growth. Creating a system for consistently reviewing relevant literature, even just a short article each week, can make a considerable impact over time. I find that dedicated time each week, even just 30 minutes, to review journals or online resources is crucial. This regular review keeps me informed of subtle changes in protocols, new research findings, and critical updates.

Staying current with medical advances and protocols demands a significant investment of time and effort. It's not a passive activity but an ongoing process requiring constant vigilance and a genuine commitment to lifelong learning. It's about cultivating a culture of inquisitiveness, critically evaluating information, and thoughtfully integrating new knowledge into practice. But the rewards are substantial: improved patient outcomes, enhanced professional skills, and increased personal fulfillment. The paramedic profession, with its dynamic and challenging nature, demands this ongoing commitment. It's an investment that ultimately benefits both the paramedic and, most importantly, the patients we serve. The sense of professional satisfaction that comes from providing the best possible care, informed by the latest medical advances, is immeasurable. It's the driving force behind my own commitment to continuing education and ongoing professional development – a commitment I urge all my colleagues to embrace with equal fervor. The lives we save, and the quality of care we provide, depend on it.

The foundation of competent paramedic practice rests upon a commitment to continuous learning, but the path to professional excellence extends beyond basic continuing education units (CEUs). Advanced training and certifications offer paramedics the opportunity to specialize, deepen their expertise, and significantly enhance their capabilities. These specialized pathways aren't just about adding letters after one's name; they represent a profound commitment to mastering complex skills and taking on greater responsibility within the dynamic landscape of prehospital care.

One of the most sought-after advanced certifications is that of a Critical Care Paramedic (CCP). This designation signifies a paramedic who has completed rigorous training in advanced life support, encompassing the management of critically ill and injured patients requiring a higher level of intervention. CCP programs typically delve into advanced airway management techniques, including the use of sophisticated ventilators and advanced airway adjuncts. They also cover hemodynamic monitoring and management, with a comprehensive understanding of cardiovascular physiology and the use of advanced medications to manage shock, cardiac arrhythmias, and other critical conditions. Furthermore, CCPs receive extensive training in the interpretation of various diagnostic modalities, including electrocardiograms (ECGs) and point-of-care ultrasound, enabling them to make more informed decisions in the field. The ability to rapidly and effectively interpret these diagnostic tools can be a true game-changer, leading to more precise and timely interventions.

I recall a particularly challenging case involving a patient experiencing severe traumatic shock. As the lead paramedic, having the CCP certification allowed me to utilize advanced hemodynamic monitoring techniques, instantly assessing the severity of the patient's condition and making informed decisions regarding fluid resuscitation and medication administration. My advanced understanding of physiology, honed through my CCP training, allowed me to anticipate potential complications and adjust treatment accordingly, ultimately contributing to a more positive patient outcome. In that instance, the extra layer of knowledge and specialized skills provided by my CCP certification proved invaluable. It was far more than just another line on a resume; it was the difference between competent care and truly exceptional patient care.

The path to becoming a Flight Paramedic (FP) is another example of advanced specialization that demands an exceptional level of skill and commitment. Flight paramedics work in demanding and often precarious environments, providing advanced life support in air medical transport. Their training encompasses not only the critical care aspects of paramedicine but also specialized knowledge in aeromedical operations, including the understanding of aircraft limitations and safety procedures. Flight paramedics must be capable of providing critical care under challenging circumstances, including altitude variations and potentially adverse weather conditions.

The challenges inherent in flight paramedicine are significant. The confined space of an aircraft often necessitates working in close proximity to other crew members while simultaneously managing the care of a critically ill patient. The constant motion of the aircraft can make simple tasks more challenging and require a degree of spatial awareness and adaptability. The need to make crucial decisions with limited resources and potentially unstable conditions demands a level of expertise and professionalism that sets flight paramedics apart. Moreover, the inherent risks associated with air medical transport, including weather hazards and mechanical failures, demand a heightened awareness of safety protocols and the ability to respond effectively to unexpected events.

Beyond critical care and flight paramedicine, a spectrum of advanced certifications exists to cater to diverse interests and career aspirations. These may include certifications in areas such as:

Pediatric Advanced Life Support (PALS): Focusing on the unique needs of critically ill and injured children. PALS certification equips paramedics with the knowledge and skills to effectively manage pediatric emergencies, taking into account the physiological differences between children and adults. This often includes specialized intubation techniques, medication dosing, and the specific challenges in treating pediatric trauma.

Neonatal Resuscitation Program (NRP): Specializing in the resuscitation and stabilization of newborns. NRP certification is crucial for paramedics working in hospitals, birthing centers, or areas where they may encounter newborns requiring immediate medical intervention. The skills and knowledge gained through NRP certification are essential for providing the delicate and life-saving care required for this vulnerable population.

Tactical Emergency Medical Services (TEMS): This specialization focuses on medical care in high-risk environments, such as active shooter situations or natural disasters. TEMS paramedics receive extensive training in working alongside law enforcement and other emergency responders, utilizing tactical approaches to ensure patient safety and effective medical interventions within hostile environments.

Disaster Management: Training in large-scale disaster response and management, providing paramedics with skills in triage, mass casualty incident management, and strategic resource allocation. Disaster management certifications equip paramedics to effectively lead and manage response efforts during large-scale emergencies, ensuring the coordination of care and resources within a chaotic and often overwhelming environment.

The acquisition of these advanced certifications not only enhances individual skills and knowledge but also significantly increases marketability and career advancement opportunities. Many EMS systems offer higher compensation and leadership positions to paramedics with advanced certifications. These certifications demonstrate a commitment to professional excellence and a desire to provide the highest level of patient care. Furthermore, they can unlock opportunities to work in specialized units or roles, such as critical care transport teams, flight programs, or hospital-based emergency departments.

However, the pursuit of advanced training and certifications is not without its challenges. The time commitment required for these programs can be significant, often demanding substantial dedication outside of regular work hours. Financial considerations also play a role, as many advanced certifications require substantial investments in tuition, course materials, and travel expenses. The rigorous nature of these programs requires dedication, discipline, and a genuine passion for the paramedic profession.

Despite these challenges, the benefits of pursuing advanced training and certifications far outweigh the obstacles. The enhanced skills and knowledge acquired translate directly into improved patient outcomes, increased job satisfaction, and greater career opportunities. Furthermore, the ongoing learning and professional development inherent in these pursuits contribute to a sense of fulfillment and ongoing professional growth. The acquisition of advanced certifications represents more than just the attainment of credentials; it's a statement about commitment to excellence and dedication to the art and science of paramedicine. It's a path towards mastery of the craft, and it's a journey I wholeheartedly recommend to any paramedic looking to further elevate their skills and impact. It's an investment in yourself, your career, and ultimately, the patients you serve. The ongoing evolution of paramedicine demands this type of proactive and dedicated approach; it's not just about keeping up, but about actively shaping the future of pre-hospital care.

Professional development extends far beyond the structured learning of advanced certifications. Regular attendance at workshops and conferences plays a crucial role in maintaining a sharp edge and staying abreast of evolving practices within the dynamic field of paramedicine. These events aren't merely opportunities for CEUs; they're vital for networking, sharing experiences, and learning from the collective wisdom of the profession.

I remember my first national paramedic conference vividly. The sheer scale of it—the buzzing energy of hundreds of paramedics, nurses, physicians, and other EMS professionals all gathered to share their knowledge and experiences—was overwhelming, yet exhilarating. It was a stark contrast to the often solitary nature of our work in the field. Suddenly, I wasn't just a single paramedic grappling with the daily challenges of the job; I was part of a vast, interconnected network of professionals, all facing similar issues and finding innovative solutions.

The workshops offered were remarkably diverse. One year, I attended a session on the latest advancements in point-of-care ultrasound.

The presenter, a renowned trauma surgeon, demonstrated techniques far beyond what I had learned during my CCP training. The detailed discussion of how to identify a pericardial effusion using ultrasound, and how to interpret that finding in the context of patient presentation, fundamentally changed my approach to assessing trauma patients. I immediately started integrating these new techniques into my practice, making my assessments far more precise and informed.

Another year, I participated in a workshop on effective communication and de-escalation techniques. This session felt particularly relevant after a particularly emotionally draining week. I had a few calls that involved significant family conflict or high emotional distress for the patients. The techniques presented—active listening, empathy, non-verbal cues, and strategies for managing conflict—proved invaluable in improving not only patient care, but also my overall ability to handle stressful situations. The insights shared during that workshop directly translated into improved patient outcomes and reduced my own stress levels in subsequent calls.

The networking aspect of these conferences is equally important. The informal conversations during coffee breaks and evening social events proved invaluable in expanding my professional network. I've formed enduring friendships and collaborations with paramedics from various parts of the country, exchanging experiences, perspectives, and insights. These connections have proved invaluable, providing invaluable peer support and facilitating professional mentorship. More than once, a connection made at a conference led to an opportunity for collaboration or even a job opening down the line.

Furthermore, conferences offer a unique opportunity to engage with industry leaders, researchers, and developers of new technologies and equipment. These interactions provide a firsthand look at emerging trends and advancements that could profoundly affect paramedic practice. One particularly enlightening experience involved attending a presentation on the development of a new type of portable ventilator. The discussion of its mechanics, capabilities, and potential clinical applications profoundly enhanced my understanding of the technological landscape within paramedicine. This allowed me to identify where the technology could be integrated into my existing practice, making my approach more efficient and effective.

However, attending professional development workshops and conferences does require careful planning and consideration. The cost of attendance, including travel, accommodation, and registration fees, can be substantial. Many organizations and EMS agencies offer partial or full funding, and it's worth exploring these avenues. Beyond the financial aspect, the time commitment required also needs to be considered. Missing time from work to attend conferences demands careful scheduling and potential arrangements for coverage during absence.

Despite these logistical hurdles, investing time and resources in professional development workshops and conferences is a worthwhile endeavor for any paramedic committed to providing exceptional patient care. The knowledge gained, the skills enhanced, the professional network expanded, and the fresh perspective obtained from interacting with colleagues from diverse backgrounds far outweigh any challenges involved.

Beyond the formal workshops and presentations, the informal opportunities for learning and networking are equally valuable. These are the incidental interactions, conversations in the hallways and during meals, where ideas are exchanged, and the unspoken nuances of the profession are shared. Often, the most profound moments of learning and self-reflection occur during these moments of casual conversation with fellow paramedics.

The evolution of paramedicine is a continuous process, driven by scientific advancements, technological innovations, and societal needs. Staying at the forefront of these changes requires proactive engagement with continuing education and professional development opportunities. Therefore, a commitment to attending workshops and conferences isn't simply a box to be checked; it's a continuous investment in the ongoing refinement of skills and knowledge. It's a dedication to a never-ending education in a dynamic field where excellence in patient care requires ongoing learning and refinement.

To maximize the benefits of these events, it's crucial to approach them strategically. Reviewing the conference agenda ahead of time and selecting workshops relevant to one's area of practice and personal development goals is essential. Actively participating in discussions, asking questions, and engaging with speakers and other attendees helps to solidify new knowledge and foster valuable connections. Afterwards, taking time to review notes, reflect on key learnings, and apply new insights into the daily practice of paramedicine is paramount for sustaining the benefits.

Furthermore, engaging with the broader EMS community through online forums, professional organizations, and social media provides valuable support, additional learning opportunities, and a constant stream of updates on new developments within the field. These digital platforms offer a means to keep abreast of breakthroughs, share experiences, and remain connected with the ever-evolving world of emergency medical services.

In conclusion, while advanced certifications represent a significant step in professional development, the regular engagement with the broader EMS community through workshops and conferences is equally crucial. These events provide a dynamic environment for learning, networking, and staying at the cutting edge of paramedicine. The time and resources invested in attending these events are a commitment to excellence, an investment in oneself, and ultimately, a crucial contribution to the improvement of patient care. The ongoing commitment to learning is not just about maintaining competence; it's about continually striving for excellence in a field that demands it.

However, the structured learning environment of workshops and conferences represents only one facet of continuous professional development. The truly dedicated paramedic understands the critical role of self-directed learning – a proactive and personalized approach to expanding knowledge and skills beyond the confines of formal training. This is where the true mastery of the profession lies: the unwavering commitment to self-improvement, fuelled by an insatiable curiosity and a desire to constantly refine one's practice.

This self-directed learning journey begins with identifying personal learning gaps and setting specific, measurable, achievable, relevant, and time-bound (SMART) goals. Reflect on recent calls. Were there any situations where you felt unprepared or uncertain about your actions? Did a particular patient presentation challenge your existing knowledge base? These reflective moments form the foundation for identifying areas requiring further study. For example, I distinctly recall a challenging case involving a patient with a complex cardiac arrhythmia. While I successfully stabilized the patient, the experience highlighted a gap in my understanding of advanced cardiac life support (ACLS) algorithms in the context of specific arrhythmias. This realization directly fuelled my decision to dedicate time to self-directed learning in this area.

Fortunately, numerous resources exist to facilitate this self-directed growth. Online learning platforms have revolutionized access to education, offering a vast array of courses, webinars, and lectures covering virtually every aspect of paramedicine. Platforms like Coursera, edX, and various EMS-specific online learning portals provide high-quality content, often delivered by leading experts in the field. The flexibility of online learning is particularly appealing to busy paramedics, allowing for asynchronous learning tailored to individual schedules. I've personally found online modules on critical care transport and prehospital pharmacology invaluable in enhancing my clinical skills and knowledge base. The convenience of accessing these resources at my own pace, fitting study sessions around my shifts and personal commitments, made a significant difference.

Beyond online courses, professional journals and publications represent an indispensable resource for self-directed learning. Journals such as *Prehospital Emergency Care, Emergency Medical Journal*, and *Resuscitation* provide peer-reviewed research, case studies, and clinical updates that keep paramedics informed about the latest advancements in the field. Regularly scanning these journals, focusing on articles relevant to one's area of interest or identified learning gaps, ensures a constant stream of fresh knowledge and insights. It's important to develop a critical eye when reviewing research, paying attention to methodology and limitations, to ensure responsible application of findings into practice.

Professional organizations, such as the National Association of Emergency Medical Technicians (NAEMT) and local EMS associations, provide a wealth of resources, including guidelines, best practices, and continuing education opportunities. Membership in these organizations offers access to exclusive content, webinars, and networking opportunities with other paramedics, fostering a sense of community and shared learning. I've found the NAEMT's PHTLS (Prehospital Trauma Life Support) course, coupled with active participation in their online forums, to be immensely valuable for maintaining proficiency in trauma management. The shared experiences and insights from fellow members are invaluable assets in personal development.

Books, too, remain a significant source of knowledge, offering in-depth exploration of specific topics within paramedicine. While online resources provide concise updates, books delve deeper, providing the context and background essential for a comprehensive understanding of complex subjects. Choosing books written by experienced paramedics and medical professionals ensures accurate and credible information. I've often found myself revisiting key texts throughout my career, gaining fresh perspectives and renewed understanding upon each rereading. This constant revisiting allows me to integrate new knowledge and learnings, continually refining my comprehension and application.

Beyond formal resources, self-directed learning involves actively seeking out opportunities for mentorship and peer learning. Engaging with senior paramedics, physicians, and nurses, asking questions, and seeking guidance on challenging cases fosters both professional growth and a stronger understanding of the clinical landscape. Likewise, connecting with peers allows for the exchange of experiences, perspectives, and practical tips—an invaluable aspect of collaborative professional development. These relationships offer a different type of learning experience. It's an exchange of practical wisdom, shaped by collective experiences, rather than a standardized course curriculum.

This process of self-directed learning is not solely an intellectual pursuit. It's a continuous cycle of reflection, action, and refinement. After completing an online course or reading a journal article, take time to reflect on the new information. Consider how it might apply to your current practice, and actively seek opportunities to integrate these new skills and knowledge into real-world situations. This continuous feedback loop, where theory is tested and refined through practice, is paramount for sustained professional development.

Moreover, the development of strong self-reflection habits is crucial for effective self-directed learning. Regularly reviewing past calls, analyzing successes and challenges, and identifying areas for improvement is a continuous process of self-assessment and growth. Journaling, whether through formal notes or informal reflections, can be a powerful tool for processing experiences and identifying patterns of behaviour or practice. Keeping a journal of clinical cases with reflections on management allows you to track your personal progress and pinpoint areas where additional training or expertise might be beneficial. These reflections can even form the basis for identifying topics for future self-directed learning initiatives.

Crucially, self-directed learning shouldn't be perceived as an isolated activity; it's deeply intertwined with overall well-being. Burnout and compassion fatigue are significant concerns in the paramedic profession, and self-care is fundamental for maintaining a sustainable career. Therefore, self-directed learning should incorporate strategies for stress management and emotional well-being. This might include exploring mindfulness techniques, engaging in physical activity, or pursuing personal hobbies as a means of balancing the demanding nature of the job. The holistic integration of self-care into the learning process ensures that the journey of professional development is not just about knowledge acquisition, but also about the preservation of physical and mental health.

In conclusion, self-directed learning is an essential component of sustained professional growth for paramedics. It's a journey fuelled by curiosity, reflection, and a commitment to continuous improvement. By utilizing the various resources available, incorporating self-reflection into practice, and prioritizing self-care, paramedics can embark on a path of self-directed learning that not only enhances their professional skills but also contributes to their overall well-being. This ongoing commitment to growth is not merely a professional responsibility; it's a personal commitment to providing the highest quality of care and maintaining a rewarding and fulfilling career in a demanding and ever-evolving field. The ongoing pursuit of knowledge and self-improvement is a constant reaffirmation of the paramedic's dedication to their patients and the profession itself. It's a journey of continuous growth that extends far beyond the classroom and the formal training setting, shaping the paramedic into a more skilled, compassionate, and resilient professional.

14

Resources and Support Networks for Paramedics

The relentless pace of emergency response, the constant exposure to trauma, and the emotional weight of life-and-death situations can leave even the most resilient paramedic feeling isolated and overwhelmed. While formal training and self-directed learning equip us with the technical skills and knowledge necessary to navigate the complexities of the job, they often fail to address the profound emotional toll. This is where the invaluable role of peer support groups comes into play. They offer a crucial lifeline, a sanctuary where paramedics can connect with colleagues who truly understand the unique challenges of the profession.

My own experience underscores the critical importance of this support network. Early in my career, I found myself grappling with a particularly difficult case involving a young child. The emotional aftermath was significant, leaving me feeling drained and questioning my ability to cope. While I had access to resources like Employee Assistance Programs (EAPs), I found the most solace and healing in conversations with experienced colleagues within my peer support group. Sharing my experience, listening to their stories, and feeling the shared weight of the profession offered a level of understanding that no formal program could replicate. It wasn't about seeking solutions; it was about validation and shared experience. It was about knowing I wasn't alone.

Peer support groups are not simply gripe sessions; they are structured environments designed to foster empathy, understanding, and a sense of shared community. They provide a safe and confidential space for paramedics to process their experiences, share coping mechanisms, and gain insights from colleagues who have navigated similar challenges. This shared experience is invaluable; it transcends the clinical realm, touching upon the emotional, psychological, and even spiritual aspects of the profession. The camaraderie fostered within these groups provides a sense of belonging, mitigating the feelings of isolation that can be so pervasive in the demanding world of emergency medical services.

The format of peer support groups can vary considerably. Some are formally organized, with designated facilitators and structured meetings. Others are more informal, evolving organically through shared experiences and professional networks. Regardless of their structure, the core function remains consistent: providing a space for open and honest communication among colleagues. This can involve sharing challenging calls, discussing ethical dilemmas, or simply venting frustrations about the pressures of the job. The emphasis is on active listening, empathy, and mutual support, creating an environment where vulnerability is not a weakness but a strength.

One particularly effective approach involves utilizing a peer-to-peer mentoring model within the group. More experienced paramedics can offer guidance and support to newer members, sharing their wisdom and experiences to help them navigate the early stages of their careers. This mentoring relationship extends beyond simply providing professional advice; it cultivates a sense of belonging and fosters a supportive network within the profession. This mentoring relationship builds upon existing trust, fostering a sense of mentorship that's deeply personal and professional.

The benefits of peer support extend beyond the immediate emotional relief they provide. They can also serve as a powerful tool for professional development. By sharing experiences and best practices, paramedics can learn from each other, expanding their clinical knowledge and refining their skills. Discussions about challenging cases can uncover different approaches to patient care, ultimately leading to improved outcomes. Moreover, the opportunity to discuss ethical dilemmas and complex clinical situations in a supportive environment fosters critical thinking and enhances decision-making skills. These discussions are not about assigning blame but about exploring different perspectives and enhancing professional judgment.

Beyond clinical knowledge, peer support groups also contribute to improved resilience and overall well-being. The ability to share vulnerabilities and receive unwavering support from colleagues strengthens the paramedic's ability to cope with stress and trauma. This emotional support acts as a buffer against burnout, compassion fatigue, and the development of Post-Traumatic Stress Disorder (PTSD). Regular participation in these groups cultivates resilience, equipping paramedics with the emotional resources necessary to navigate the demanding nature of their profession.

Furthermore, peer support groups can play a crucial role in promoting mental health awareness and reducing the stigma associated with seeking help. The open and honest nature of these groups creates a space where paramedics feel comfortable discussing mental health concerns, reducing the sense of shame or isolation that often accompanies mental health struggles. This can encourage colleagues to seek professional help when needed, preventing mental health issues from escalating into more serious problems.

However, the effectiveness of peer support groups hinges on several key factors. Confidentiality is paramount; members must trust that their disclosures will be respected and remain within the group. A strong sense of mutual respect and empathy is also crucial, creating an environment where members feel comfortable being vulnerable. The group should be facilitated by someone with training in trauma-informed care and mental health, ensuring the conversations are guided in a safe and supportive manner. In my experience, groups without experienced facilitators often flounder, falling into unproductive venting rather than focused support and problem-solving.

The establishment and maintenance of peer support groups often require the proactive involvement of EMS agencies and professional organizations. Providing resources, training, and dedicated space for these groups is crucial in ensuring their success and accessibility to all paramedics. A well-structured program may include training sessions on effective communication techniques, active listening, and boundaries in peer-to-peer support. This provides a framework for constructive conversation that transcends casual chats. Agency support also acknowledges the vital role these groups play in workforce wellness, reinforcing the value of mental and emotional health within the organization. This institutional support is not just about providing resources, it's also about demonstrating a commitment to the well-being of the paramedics themselves.

In conclusion, peer support groups offer an indispensable resource for paramedics, providing a safe space to connect with colleagues, share experiences, and offer mutual support. They represent more than just a source of emotional comfort; they are a vital component of comprehensive well-being strategies for this demanding profession. By fostering camaraderie, facilitating professional development, and promoting mental health awareness, peer support groups contribute significantly to the overall resilience and effectiveness of paramedic teams. Investing in these groups is not merely a matter of employee care; it's an investment in the quality of patient care, professional excellence, and the longevity of the paramedic workforce. The strength of a profession is built not just on individual capabilities, but on the interwoven support and understanding that binds its members together. The dedication to building and maintaining these vital support systems is a testament to a profession's commitment to its own well-being and, ultimately, the well-being of the communities it serves.

The shared support of peer groups provides an invaluable first step in addressing the mental health challenges faced by paramedics, but it's crucial to recognize its limitations. Peer support, while incredibly beneficial for camaraderie and initial emotional processing, cannot replace the expertise of trained mental health professionals. Just as we rely on specialized medical professionals for physical injuries, we need to embrace the same approach to our mental and emotional well-being. This necessitates actively seeking and engaging with mental health professionals who specialize in the unique trauma experienced by first responders.

The stigma surrounding mental health within the profession remains a significant barrier. Many paramedics, deeply ingrained with a culture of stoicism and self-reliance, hesitate to seek help, fearing judgment, career repercussions, or the perception of weakness. This silence perpetuates a cycle of suffering, preventing individuals from accessing the care they desperately need. I've seen this firsthand – colleagues silently struggling, masking their pain behind a facade of strength, until their burden becomes too heavy to bear. We must actively challenge this pervasive culture and cultivate an environment where seeking help is not only accepted but actively encouraged.

Finding the right mental health professional is crucial. While many therapists are compassionate and well-intentioned, not all possess the specialized understanding necessary to effectively address the complex trauma experienced by paramedics. The specific nature of our work—witnessing death, injury, violence, and suffering on a regular basis—requires a therapist who understands the unique stressors and challenges inherent in this profession. They need to understand the concept of moral injury, compassion fatigue, and the cumulative effects of prolonged exposure to trauma. A therapist unfamiliar with these concepts might misinterpret symptoms or offer ineffective treatments. This is not to diminish the value of other therapists, but to emphasize the importance of finding someone with specialized knowledge.

Therefore, actively seeking out therapists with experience in treating first responders is paramount. This can involve researching therapists online, contacting local EMS agencies or professional organizations for referrals, or speaking with colleagues who have successfully navigated this process. Many organizations now have dedicated support lines and resources specifically for first responders, often connecting individuals with therapists familiar with the unique challenges of the profession. These organizations can provide invaluable guidance and support throughout the process. Remember, this search is an investment in your well-being, and finding the right fit is crucial to the success of your therapy journey.

Once you've found a potential therapist, the initial consultation is key. During this meeting, it's vital to openly and honestly communicate your experiences, concerns, and expectations. Don't hesitate to ask about their experience working with first responders, their approach to therapy, and their understanding of the specific challenges you face. This is your opportunity to assess whether their approach aligns with your needs and whether you feel comfortable establishing a therapeutic relationship with them. A strong therapeutic alliance—built on trust, respect, and mutual understanding—is crucial for effective treatment. Trust your gut; if something doesn't feel right, don't hesitate to seek a second opinion.

The types of therapy that can be beneficial for paramedics vary, but evidence-based approaches like Cognitive Behavioral Therapy (CBT), Trauma-Focused Cognitive Behavioral Therapy (TF-CBT), and Eye Movement Desensitization and Reprocessing (EMDR) have demonstrated effectiveness in addressing trauma-related symptoms. CBT helps to identify and modify negative thought patterns and behaviors contributing to stress and anxiety. TF-CBT focuses on processing traumatic memories and developing coping mechanisms. EMDR uses bilateral stimulation to help process traumatic memories, reducing their emotional intensity. Your therapist can help determine which approach best suits your individual needs and preferences.

Beyond individual therapy, other support systems can prove invaluable. Support groups specifically for first responders offer a space to connect with others who understand the unique challenges of the profession. These groups provide a sense of community, reducing feelings of isolation and fostering mutual support. They can also be a platform for sharing coping strategies and learning from others' experiences. These aren't replacements for therapy but valuable supplemental resources. Even casual interactions with supportive colleagues can significantly impact well-being.

Furthermore, exploring complementary therapies like mindfulness practices, yoga, or meditation can enhance mental and emotional well-being. These practices can help to reduce stress, improve self-awareness, and promote emotional regulation. They are tools to integrate into your self-care routine, strengthening your resilience against burnout and trauma. These practices aren't quick fixes but sustainable methods for self-care.

The path to mental wellness is not linear, and it requires commitment and perseverance. There will be setbacks and challenges along the way, but remember that seeking help is a sign of strength, not weakness. It's an active decision to prioritize your well-being and protect your ability to continue serving your community effectively. It's a testament to your resilience and self-awareness. The commitment to your mental health should be just as valued as your commitment to physical health. It's an ongoing process of self-discovery and growth.

Many agencies now offer Employee Assistance Programs (EAPs) that provide confidential counseling services. These programs can be a good starting point for accessing mental health support. However, it's vital to remember that EAPs may have limitations in their scope of services or the level of specialized care they can offer. They are often a good first step towards connecting with a more specialized therapist.

Remember that taking care of your mental health isn't selfish; it's essential to your ability to effectively perform your duties and maintain healthy relationships. The well-being of paramedics directly impacts the quality of patient care. A burned-out, emotionally exhausted paramedic is less capable of providing optimal care. Prioritizing your mental health is not only beneficial for you but also for the communities you serve. The commitment to your mental health contributes to a more resilient, effective, and compassionate emergency response system.

Taking that first step to seek professional help can feel daunting, but remember that you are not alone. Many paramedics have successfully navigated this journey, and with the right support and resources, you can too. Reaching out is a sign of courage and a commitment to your well-being. It's an acknowledgment that self-care is a critical component of a long and fulfilling career in EMS. You deserve to receive the same level of professional care that you dedicate to your patients. It's a matter of self-preservation and maintaining a professional life that you can sustain long-term. The ability to thrive in this profession is directly linked to your well-being – taking charge of your mental health is an investment in your career and your life. Never underestimate the profound impact seeking help can have.

It's also worth remembering that your journey to mental wellness is personal and unique. What works for one paramedic may not work for another. Be patient with yourself, allow time for exploration and adjustment, and don't be afraid to try different approaches. The key is finding what helps you manage stress, process trauma, and maintain a sense of balance in your life. This is a journey of self-discovery and healing. It's a commitment to your well-being – both now and in the long term.

Finally, remember that seeking help is not a sign of failure; it is a testament to your strength and your commitment to your well-being. It shows that you value your mental health and are committed to thriving in your demanding profession. Your well-being is just as vital as your technical skills, and investing in your mental health is an investment in the success of your career and your personal life. Remember that the strength of the EMS profession isn't just found in the skills and technical proficiency of its members, but also in the strength and resilience of the individuals themselves.

Many agencies now offer Employee Assistance Programs (EAPs) as a vital component of their employee benefits packages. These programs are designed to provide confidential support and resources to employees struggling with a wide range of personal and professional challenges, including those unique to the demanding world of emergency medical services. While EAPs aren't a replacement for dedicated mental health care, they often serve as a crucial first step toward accessing support and identifying the most appropriate path forward.

The services offered by EAPs can vary significantly depending on the agency and the provider they contract with. However, common services frequently include short-term counseling, access to a network of mental health professionals, and resources for stress management techniques. Some EAPs may even extend their services to include legal and financial consultations, recognizing that financial worries and legal issues can significantly contribute to overall stress and well-being.

One of the most significant advantages of EAPs is their confidentiality. Employees can access these services without fear of repercussions within their workplace. This confidentiality is essential for fostering open communication and encouraging employees to seek help without hesitation. The anonymity offered by EAPs breaks down the stigma often associated with seeking mental health support, empowering individuals to prioritize their well-being without concerns about potential judgments or career impacts. This is especially crucial within the EMS profession, where the culture of stoicism can sometimes hinder help-seeking behavior.

My experience working with paramedics has highlighted the importance of easily accessible, confidential resources. I recall one instance where a colleague, struggling with post-traumatic stress following a particularly harrowing call, initially hesitated to seek professional help due to fear of stigmatization. He was only comfortable discussing his experiences after learning about the agency's EAP and the safeguards in place to protect his privacy. This experience underscores the vital role of EAPs in breaking down barriers and promoting mental health awareness. The EAP provided him with a safe space to begin processing his trauma, eventually leading him to seek more extensive therapy.

However, it's important to acknowledge the limitations of EAPs. The services are often limited to a specific number of sessions, and the focus is usually on short-term interventions rather than long-term therapy. While this initial support can be incredibly valuable for addressing immediate concerns and stabilizing a crisis, it might not suffice for managing complex trauma or chronic mental health issues. Think of an EAP as a first responder in the realm of mental health – it provides immediate assistance and can help identify the next steps needed.

The type of support offered can also be limited. While stress management and coping skills workshops are invaluable, they often lack the depth of personalized care that a dedicated therapist can provide. This is why it's critical to view EAPs as a stepping stone, not a destination. They can be an effective entry point into the mental health care system, providing a safe space to begin the conversation and begin the healing process. Many EAPs can also help connect individuals with long-term therapists specializing in the needs of first responders. This connection, made possible through the initial support of the EAP, can be invaluable in ensuring ongoing, tailored care.

Furthermore, the quality of EAP services can vary significantly depending on the provider. It is crucial to explore the available services within your agency's EAP to determine what resources are available. Understanding the scope of services – such as the number of sessions offered, the types of therapists available, and any limitations on the types of issues addressed – is a necessary step in effectively utilizing the program. Don't hesitate to ask questions and advocate for yourself to ensure that the EAP appropriately meets your needs.

Beyond direct counseling services, many EAPs offer valuable resources like educational materials on stress management, work-life balance, and coping mechanisms. These resources can be particularly beneficial for paramedics struggling to navigate the emotional and physical demands of their profession. Access to online self-help modules, webinars, or workbooks can complement counseling sessions by providing ongoing support and tools for self-management.

The integration of EAPs within the organizational culture of an EMS agency is equally crucial for its success. If the agency actively promotes the use of EAP services and demonstrates a commitment to employee well-being, it's more likely that employees will feel comfortable utilizing these resources. Leadership's visible support of mental health initiatives, coupled with clear communication about the availability and benefits of EAPs, can significantly impact its utilization.

In my experience, I've witnessed the profound positive impact of agencies that actively champion the use of EAPs. When a culture of support is fostered, where seeking help is normalized and encouraged rather than stigmatized, employees are more likely to proactively engage with the available resources. This creates a supportive work environment where employees feel valued and prioritize their mental well-being.

However, even with a supportive agency culture, some paramedics may still hesitate to reach out to EAPs. This hesitation might stem from individual factors like previous negative experiences with mental health services, mistrust, or the deeply ingrained belief that seeking help constitutes a sign of weakness. Addressing these underlying barriers requires a multifaceted approach that encompasses increased education, open dialogue, and a leadership commitment to fostering a supportive and inclusive work environment.

It's imperative that agencies ensure their EAPs are culturally sensitive and offer services that are accessible to all employees, regardless of background, language, or cultural beliefs. This includes having multilingual support, culturally competent therapists, and readily available information about available services in various formats.

In conclusion, Employee Assistance Programs offer a crucial lifeline for paramedics navigating the emotional and psychological challenges inherent to their demanding profession. While EAPs are not a panacea, they serve as an invaluable first step towards accessing support and fostering a culture of mental wellness within EMS agencies. By understanding their strengths and limitations, actively promoting their use, and ensuring that these programs are accessible and comprehensive, we can significantly improve the well-being of the brave men and women who serve on the front lines of emergency medical care. The success of EAPs hinges on a combined effort – the agency's proactive support, the individual's willingness to seek help, and the provision of easily accessible and high-quality resources. Ultimately, a focus on mental health within the EMS community is an investment in a stronger, more resilient, and ultimately more effective emergency response system. The well-being of our paramedics is not just a matter of individual health; it's a matter of public safety and community welfare.

Beyond the immediate support offered by individual agencies through EAPs, a wider network of governmental and non-profit organizations provides crucial resources and support for paramedics. These external resources often offer a broader scope of services and can fill gaps in support not covered by internal agency programs. Understanding these resources is critical for paramedics seeking help, and for agencies striving to support their workforce holistically.

One significant area where external organizations play a vital role is mental health support. The cumulative stress and trauma inherent in paramedic work often lead to mental health challenges like PTSD, depression, and anxiety. While EAPs provide a crucial initial point of contact, many paramedics find themselves needing more extensive, long-term therapeutic intervention. This is where specialized organizations dedicated to first responders' mental health become invaluable. These organizations often provide specialized therapy tailored to the unique stressors faced by emergency medical personnel, utilizing evidence-based treatments such as prolonged exposure therapy, cognitive processing therapy, and eye movement desensitization and reprocessing (EMDR). They also frequently offer peer support programs, connecting paramedics with others who understand the challenges of the profession and can offer empathy and understanding. The sense of community and shared experience can be profoundly therapeutic. These organizations may offer group therapy sessions, workshops focused on stress management and resilience-building techniques, and even retreats designed for rest and recovery.

The availability and nature of these organizations vary by geographic location. Some are national organizations with a broad reach, while others operate regionally or even locally, catering to specific communities or regions. It's essential for paramedics to research organizations within their area to identify relevant resources. Many national organizations maintain websites with directories or search tools, facilitating the discovery of local support networks. A simple internet search for "first responder mental health support [your state/province/country]" is an excellent starting point.

Financial aid is another critical area where external support can make a significant difference. Paramedics, like many other professions, face financial strains that can compound the stress of the job. Unexpected medical bills, family emergencies, or even career interruptions can quickly destabilize finances. Several non-profit organizations provide financial assistance to first responders facing financial hardship. These organizations often offer grants, loans, or emergency financial aid to help paramedics cover essential expenses. The eligibility criteria and application processes vary significantly across organizations, so it's crucial to research specific organizations to understand their requirements. These organizations often have strict guidelines and prioritize individuals demonstrating a clear need. The application process frequently involves providing extensive documentation, outlining financial need and the circumstances leading to the need for assistance. Building a supportive network of individuals and organizations familiar with your situation can be invaluable during this process.

Beyond mental health and financial assistance, some governmental and non-profit organizations offer additional crucial resources. These may include legal aid services for paramedics facing legal challenges related to their work, educational opportunities for professional development or career advancement, and resources for work-life balance support. Some organizations focus on providing training and resources regarding ethical dilemmas, helping paramedics navigate complex situations involving patient care, agency protocols, and legal responsibilities. Others offer career transition services for paramedics seeking to change careers or retire from the demanding profession. Understanding the spectrum of services available can empower paramedics to proactively address diverse needs and challenges. These resources often exist in tandem with mental health support, recognizing that financial stability and career contentment can significantly contribute to improved mental well-being.

It's also important to acknowledge the limitations of these external support organizations. Funding often restricts the scale of services they can offer, and wait times for appointments or financial aid can sometimes be lengthy. The criteria for eligibility can be stringent, requiring individuals to meet specific qualifications to access support. The rigorous application processes, while necessary for responsible distribution of resources, can be disheartening for those in crisis. Therefore, it's crucial to be persistent and persistent and to explore all available avenues. Networking with peers and colleagues can help paramedics discover hidden resources and navigate the application processes effectively. Support groups offer a valuable avenue for sharing information, learning about successful strategies for accessing aid, and fostering a sense of community among those facing shared struggles.

Building a relationship with a social worker or case manager experienced in working with first responders can be extremely valuable. They can often assist in navigating the complexities of the system, connecting paramedics with relevant organizations, and providing guidance throughout the application process. These professionals understand the unique challenges faced by paramedics and can advocate for individuals' needs. They can also act as a liaison between the paramedic and the organizations providing support, streamlining communication and ensuring timely access to services. Their expertise in navigating bureaucratic processes can significantly reduce the stress and burden associated with obtaining support. They can also help paramedics understand the implications of various services and choose the options most suited to their individual needs.

Furthermore, many governmental agencies have initiatives designed to improve the health and well-being of first responders. These initiatives can range from public awareness campaigns to educational programs promoting mental health awareness and stress management. Some governments fund research into the specific challenges faced by first responders and develop evidence-based interventions to address these issues. Staying informed about these initiatives can provide paramedics with valuable resources and highlight the importance of prioritizing their well-being.

In closing, while EAPs offer an essential first line of support, the broader network of government and non-profit organizations provides a vital complement. These organizations offer specialized services, broader resources, and expanded support for paramedics navigating the complex challenges of their profession. It's crucial for paramedics to proactively research available resources, understand their eligibility criteria, and develop a support network to help them access and utilize these vital services. By understanding the available support systems and building a strong support network, paramedics can better manage the stresses of their profession and ensure their long-term well-being. The act of actively seeking support is a testament to strength and resilience, not a sign of weakness. It's a critical step in safeguarding the health and welfare of those who dedicate their lives to serving their communities. Investing in the well-being of paramedics is an investment in a stronger, more resilient, and more effective emergency response system.

The previous sections highlighted the crucial role of formal support systems—EAPs and external organizations—in bolstering the well-being of paramedics. However, the support network extends far beyond these structured channels. The digital age has fostered a unique and invaluable resource: online communities and forums specifically designed for paramedics. These virtual spaces offer a sense of connection, camaraderie, and shared understanding that can be profoundly impactful on mental health and professional development. They're a lifeline for many, offering a level of support that's both immediate and readily accessible, regardless of location or time of day.

My own experience highlights the power of these online networks. During a particularly challenging period in my career—a period involving a series of traumatic calls that left me emotionally depleted—I stumbled upon a paramedic forum. At first, I was hesitant. The idea of sharing my vulnerabilities online felt exposed, even risky. But the anonymity offered by the platform, coupled with the overwhelming sense of shared experience, encouraged me to participate. What I found was a community of individuals who understood the unique pressures of the job, the moral ambiguities, and the emotional toll. The simple act of reading others' posts, acknowledging their struggles, and sharing my own experiences without judgment proved to be incredibly cathartic. It was a virtual safe space where I could freely express my emotions without the fear of judgment or repercussions. The advice and support I received, from coping mechanisms to career navigation, were invaluable during that difficult period.

These online spaces serve as more than just a platform for venting frustrations or sharing war stories. They offer a rich tapestry of support, connecting paramedics across geographical boundaries and diverse experiences. Think of a paramedic in rural Montana grappling with isolation, finding solace in the shared experiences of a paramedic working in the bustling emergency room of a major city hospital in New York. The ability to connect with others who understand the nuances of the profession, regardless of their specific context, is a powerful antidote to feelings of isolation and professional alienation.

The nature of these online communities is diverse. Some are tightly knit, closed groups, requiring membership applications and often fostering a high level of trust and confidentiality. Others are more open forums, allowing for broader participation but possibly sacrificing some level of intimate support. Some are hosted on dedicated professional platforms, offering curated resources and moderated discussions, while others exist on more general social media sites, relying on self-regulation and the collective wisdom of the community.

Regardless of their structure, these online communities often function as a decentralized system of support. They offer opportunities for:

Peer Support: This is perhaps the most valuable aspect of these online communities. The ability to connect with fellow paramedics who understand the emotional and physical demands of the job provides a powerful sense of validation and belonging. Sharing experiences, both positive and negative, fosters a sense of solidarity and mutual support. Knowing that you're not alone in your struggles, that others have faced similar challenges and overcome them, is a profound source of strength and resilience.

Information Sharing: These online forums often become repositories of knowledge and expertise. Paramedics share best practices, discuss challenging cases, and debate ethical dilemmas. This exchange of information is invaluable for professional development, keeping paramedics updated on the latest advancements in emergency medicine and providing a platform for continuous learning. The collective wisdom of the community can be a powerful tool for enhancing skills and improving patient care.

Mental Health Support: Beyond peer support, many online communities provide a space for discussing mental health challenges. Paramedics often feel hesitant to discuss these issues with their supervisors or colleagues face-to-face, but the relative anonymity of an online forum can encourage open dialogue. Sharing experiences with others who understand the specific mental health challenges faced by first responders can be incredibly helpful in managing stress, anxiety, and trauma. Discussions around coping mechanisms, therapy resources, and self-care strategies are common within these communities.

Networking and Career Development: Online forums can be excellent tools for networking and career advancement. Paramedics can connect with colleagues from other agencies, explore career opportunities, and seek advice on professional development. Discussions about continuing education, advanced certifications, and career transitions are frequent occurrences within these communities. The ability to tap into a vast network of professionals can open up unforeseen possibilities.

Advocacy and Activism: Online communities can serve as platforms for collective action. Paramedics can unite to advocate for improved working conditions, better pay, and enhanced mental health resources. They can share information about legislation affecting the profession and organize efforts to bring about positive change. The collective voice of paramedics, amplified through these online networks, can have a significant impact on policy and practice.

However, it's crucial to acknowledge the limitations of online support networks. The information shared online shouldn't replace professional medical advice. While these communities offer a powerful sense of connection, they should not be the sole source of support. The anonymity of the internet can also harbor risks, including misinformation and potentially harmful interactions. It is essential to approach these online spaces with a critical eye, verifying information and being mindful of personal safety. Furthermore, the online environment can sometimes exacerbate feelings of isolation if not navigated responsibly. Consistent engagement with real-world support systems—friends, family, and professional help—remains essential.

Finally, building a robust support network requires a multifaceted approach. While online communities provide invaluable support, they should be integrated with, not replace, the formal support structures already discussed. The ideal scenario is a synergistic blend of structured organizational support and the informal, dynamic support offered by online communities. This holistic approach acknowledges the individual needs of paramedics, recognizing that effective coping mechanisms often require a combination of formal and informal, personal and professional support systems. The judicious use of online communities, coupled with engagement with EAPs, external organizations, and personal support networks, provides a comprehensive strategy for nurturing mental well-being and ensuring long-term resilience within this demanding profession. The strength of a paramedic's support network is directly proportional to their ability to navigate the complexities of the job and sustain a fulfilling career. Building this network, both online and offline, is an essential act of self-care and professional stewardship.

15

The Future of Paramedicine

The integration of technology into emergency medical services (EMS) is no longer a futuristic fantasy; it's a rapidly evolving reality reshaping the landscape of prehospital care. This transformation, driven by advancements in telecommunications, artificial intelligence (AI), and data analytics, promises to revolutionize how we respond to emergencies, diagnose conditions, and ultimately, save lives. However, this technological leap also presents complex ethical considerations that demand careful navigation.

Telehealth, for instance, is rapidly expanding the reach of paramedics beyond the confines of the ambulance. Remote consultations via video conferencing allow for real-time assessments of patients in the field, providing guidance to paramedics and potentially avoiding unnecessary transports to the emergency room. Imagine a scenario where a paramedic encounters a patient experiencing chest pain in a remote area with limited access to advanced medical facilities. Through telehealth, a cardiologist or emergency physician can remotely assess the patient's electrocardiogram (ECG), offer a preliminary diagnosis, and provide crucial instructions for management, potentially averting a potentially fatal delay in treatment. This technology not only improves the quality of care but also optimizes resource allocation, reducing the strain on overcrowded emergency departments.

The applications of telehealth are surprisingly diverse. From providing crucial support to paramedics in challenging situations—think of a paramedic struggling with a complex intubation in a rural setting receiving real-time guidance from an expert—to conducting post-discharge follow-ups with patients, improving patient outcomes and satisfaction, telehealth is fundamentally transforming how we deliver prehospital care. The ability to remotely monitor vital signs, transmit images, and communicate seamlessly with specialists is drastically changing the dynamic of emergency medical response, particularly in underserved communities where access to specialized medical expertise is limited.

The rise of AI is another significant game-changer in paramedicine. AI-powered diagnostic tools are being developed that can analyze data from a variety of sources, such as ECGs, vital signs, and patient history, to provide paramedics with more accurate and timely diagnoses. These tools can assist in identifying patterns and anomalies that may be missed by the human eye, leading to earlier interventions and improved patient outcomes. Picture a scenario where an AI algorithm identifies a subtle abnormality in an ECG that indicates a potentially life-threatening arrhythmia, alerting the paramedic to the need for immediate intervention before it's too late.

Moreover, AI's ability to process vast amounts of data can help predict and prevent emergencies. By analyzing historical data on emergency calls, patient demographics, and environmental factors, AI can identify high-risk areas and populations, enabling proactive interventions and resource allocation. For example, an AI system might predict a surge in emergency calls during a heatwave, allowing EMS agencies to deploy additional resources to affected areas. This proactive approach not only improves response times but also potentially mitigates the severity of health crises. However, the reliance on AI necessitates careful consideration of data privacy and algorithmic bias. Ensuring these systems are trained on diverse and representative datasets and are transparent in their decision-making process is paramount.

Drone technology offers yet another exciting frontier in paramedicine. Drones can be used to deliver critical supplies, such as medication or blood products, to remote areas or disaster zones where access is limited. Imagine a situation where a stroke patient requires a rapid delivery of a clot-busting drug. A drone could rapidly deliver the medication, drastically reducing the time to treatment and improving the patient's chances of a full recovery. Drones could also be used for surveillance during large-scale events, assisting in search and rescue operations, and even conducting preliminary assessments of scenes before paramedics arrive. The potential applications of drones in emergency medicine are vast and continually evolving.

However, the integration of drone technology raises critical questions regarding safety, regulations, and airspace management. Ensuring the safe and efficient operation of drones in complex environments requires careful planning and coordination. The regulatory framework governing the use of drones for medical purposes needs to be robust and adaptable to the rapid pace of technological advancement.

The ethical implications of these technological advancements in paramedicine cannot be overlooked. Issues of data privacy, algorithmic bias, and the potential displacement of human paramedics require careful consideration. As AI and telehealth systems become more sophisticated, concerns about the accountability and responsibility for medical decisions arise. Maintaining the human element of care, ensuring empathy and compassion remain at the heart of the profession, even as technology increases, is crucial.

It's not just about the technologies themselves; it's about how they're integrated into the existing workflow and culture of EMS systems. The successful integration of technology requires substantial investment in training and education for paramedics. They must be equipped with the skills and knowledge to effectively use these new tools, understand their limitations, and integrate them seamlessly into their clinical practice. This involves not just technical training but also education on ethical considerations and the importance of human interaction in patient care.

Furthermore, the societal impact of these technological advancements cannot be ignored. The cost-effectiveness of telehealth and AI-powered diagnostic tools needs careful evaluation. The accessibility of these technologies needs to be equitable, ensuring that they benefit all members of society, regardless of socioeconomic status or geographic location. Any increase in efficiency or cost reduction must not come at the expense of patient safety or the erosion of the patient-paramedic relationship, which is foundational to effective and compassionate care.

In conclusion, the future of paramedicine is inextricably linked to the rapid evolution of technology. Telehealth, AI, and drone technology are poised to revolutionize prehospital care, improving the quality of care, optimizing resource allocation, and potentially saving lives. However, navigating this technological transformation requires a thoughtful approach that carefully considers the ethical implications, addresses potential biases, ensures equitable access, and prioritizes the preservation of the human element in emergency medical response. The integration of technology isn't merely about replacing human skills, but rather augmenting them, empowering paramedics to provide even better, more efficient, and more compassionate care in the face of increasingly complex medical emergencies. This balanced approach will ensure that technology serves as a tool to empower paramedics, not replace them. The future of paramedicine lies not in the replacement of humans by machines, but in the collaborative partnership between them, working together to provide the highest standard of care possible.

The shift towards value-based care, a payment model emphasizing quality over quantity, is profoundly reshaping the landscape of healthcare delivery. This paradigm shift, which prioritizes patient outcomes and cost-effectiveness, is having a direct impact on emergency medical services (EMS). Historically, EMS systems have operated under a fee-for-service model, where reimbursement was largely determined by the number of transports to the emergency department. This incentivized volume, potentially leading to unnecessary transports and placing a strain on already overburdened hospital systems. Value-based care, however, necessitates a more nuanced approach.

Under value-based care, EMS agencies are increasingly being held accountable for the overall health outcomes of their patients. This requires a shift in focus from simply transporting patients to hospitals to proactively managing their care, potentially preventing hospitalizations altogether. This involves a greater emphasis on community paramedicine, a model of care where paramedics provide a broader range of services in the community, beyond the traditional emergency response. Community paramedicine programs often include chronic disease management, preventative care visits, and post-discharge follow-up. This expansion of roles empowers paramedics to address the root causes of healthcare issues, improving patient outcomes and reducing the overall burden on hospitals.

I remember a specific case from my early years as a paramedic. We were called to an elderly woman with repeated falls. Under the old system, we would've transported her to the emergency department for evaluation, regardless of the underlying cause. However, through a community paramedicine program, I was able to conduct a thorough assessment at her home, identify that she was experiencing medication side effects, and coordinate with her physician to adjust her medication regime. This simple intervention prevented a hospital visit, alleviated her falls, and improved her quality of life. The shift to value-based care made this type of proactive intervention not just possible, but expected and often financially rewarded, incentivizing improved care pathways.

The integration of EMS into accountable care organizations (ACOs) is further accelerating this transformation. ACOs are groups of health-care providers who work together to coordinate patient care and improve overall health outcomes. By incorporating EMS into these networks, ACOs can gain a broader understanding of the patient population's needs and develop more effective strategies for disease prevention and management. This collaborative approach ensures that EMS providers are not just responding to emergencies, but actively participating in the long-term management of patients' health, optimizing patient pathways, and reducing hospital readmissions. It demands a high level of inter-professional collaboration, seamless communication, and shared clinical responsibility, all contributing to enhanced patient care and health system efficiency.

The growing emphasis on preventative care is another significant trend impacting EMS. With the rising prevalence of chronic diseases, the focus is shifting towards proactive intervention and risk reduction. This involves paramedics playing a more active role in health screenings, health education, and the identification of patients at high risk of developing serious medical conditions. For example, paramedics might conduct blood pressure screenings in community centers or schools, educating individuals on lifestyle modifications to reduce their risk of cardiovascular disease. This proactive approach not only prevents serious health crises but also reduces the overall cost of healthcare, aligning perfectly with the principles of value-based care.

However, this transformation is not without its challenges. The transition to value-based care requires a significant shift in mindset and practices within the EMS community. Paramedics are being asked to assume expanded roles that require advanced training and new skill sets. The implementation of value-based care also requires strong partnerships with other healthcare providers, seamless data sharing, and efficient communication across the healthcare continuum. Building these collaborative relationships can be complex, especially across different healthcare organizations with their unique processes and systems. Data security and patient privacy become equally important considerations, necessitating robust systems for data management and ensuring compliance with relevant regulations.

Furthermore, the financial sustainability of community paramedicine and other value-based programs remains a significant hurdle. Reimbursement models need to be sufficiently robust to support these expanded roles and compensate paramedics for their increased responsibilities. Negotiating fair reimbursement rates with payers and developing sustainable funding models are crucial for the long-term success of these programs. This necessitates a strong advocacy role for EMS agencies and professional organizations to ensure adequate financial support and fair compensation for the evolving roles and responsibilities of paramedics.

The legal and regulatory frameworks surrounding EMS also need to adapt to these changes. Expanding the scope of practice for paramedics requires clear guidelines and regulations to ensure patient safety and legal compliance. Developing and implementing these new regulations requires a collaborative effort between EMS agencies, healthcare organizations, and government bodies. This includes clear definition of scope of practice, liability protection for paramedics performing expanded roles, and transparent regulatory processes for program approval and oversight.

The transition to value-based care also necessitates a significant investment in technology and infrastructure. Telehealth platforms, electronic health records (EHRs), and data analytics tools are crucial for the efficient delivery of care and the accurate tracking of patient outcomes. Integrating these technologies into existing EMS systems can be costly and complex, requiring substantial investment and ongoing training for paramedics and support staff. Accessibility is a crucial consideration; the technological enhancements must be accessible to all, regardless of location or socioeconomic status, to ensure equity of care.

In conclusion, the changes in healthcare delivery are reshaping the role of paramedics in profound ways. The shift towards value-based care, community paramedicine, and integration into ACOs are transforming how emergency medical services are delivered and perceived. While this transformation presents significant opportunities to improve patient outcomes and enhance the efficiency of the healthcare system, navigating the financial, regulatory, and technological challenges is crucial for the long-term success of these initiatives. The future of paramedicine lies in embracing these changes, advocating for appropriate support, and continually adapting to meet the evolving needs of the healthcare system and the communities we serve. It requires ongoing professional development, strong inter-professional collaborations, and a commitment to innovation to provide efficient, equitable, and compassionate care that aligns with the principles of value-based healthcare. The ultimate goal is not simply to respond to emergencies but to actively prevent them, managing patients' overall health and well-being within their broader community context.

The escalating complexity of public health demands a multifaceted response, and paramedics, by virtue of their unique position at the intersection of healthcare and the community, are increasingly crucial players. Their front-line role affords them unparalleled insight into emerging health threats, allowing for early detection and rapid response. This is particularly evident in the wake of recent events, highlighting the need for enhanced preparedness and adaptability within the paramedic profession.

The COVID-19 pandemic dramatically underscored the vulnerabilities within our healthcare systems and the critical importance of a well-trained and resilient paramedic workforce. In the initial stages, paramedics were often the first responders to patients exhibiting symptoms, frequently facing uncertainty and a significant lack of personal protective equipment (PPE). The rapid evolution of the virus and the constantly shifting understanding of its transmission necessitated quick adaptation and training protocols. I recall a particularly harrowing early shift where we responded to a suspected COVID case with only rudimentary PPE – surgical masks and gloves – a stark reminder of the immediate and substantial challenges the pandemic imposed. The subsequent waves of the pandemic required a significant shift in our protocols, incorporating more sophisticated PPE, and specialized training in managing patients with varying levels of respiratory distress and oxygenation needs. We had to learn quickly to navigate the emotional toll of seeing so much suffering, coupled with the constant fear of contracting the virus ourselves.

The pandemic's impact highlighted the need for robust surveillance systems and effective communication networks, allowing for efficient information sharing and resource allocation. The lack of readily available testing and accurate data in the initial stages hampered the response, emphasizing the importance of rapid diagnostic tools and clear communication pathways between paramedics, hospitals, and public health authorities. Our dispatch system, usually fairly efficient, was overwhelmed in the early days. Delayed information and strained communication channels increased stress levels and hampered effective patient management. This underscored the critical need for integrated digital platforms capable of handling increased demand and providing real-time updates on resources and protocols. The experience was a sharp lesson in the importance of adaptable infrastructure and consistent, timely, and clear communication during public health crises.

Beyond pandemics, climate change poses a growing public health threat, and paramedics are on the front lines. Extreme weather events, such as heatwaves, floods, and wildfires, result in an increase in emergency calls related to heatstroke, injuries, respiratory illnesses, and mental health crises. I've personally experienced the dramatic increase in heatstroke calls during prolonged periods of intense heat. The physical and emotional demands placed on paramedics during and after such disasters are immense, as they not only provide immediate medical care, but often play a crucial role in rescue and evacuation efforts. The frequency and intensity of these events are predicted to rise, requiring proactive measures, including specialized training in disaster response, and access to advanced equipment for mitigating the effects of extreme weather.

Moreover, the growing prevalence of chronic diseases requires a proactive approach to prevention and management. Paramedics are uniquely positioned to engage in public health initiatives aimed at improving community wellness. Community paramedicine programs are increasingly important, providing paramedics with the opportunity to conduct health screenings, participate in disease management, and deliver preventative health education. This includes blood pressure and glucose screenings, education on healthy lifestyle choices, and follow-up care for chronic conditions. The expanded role of paramedics in this context requires specialized training in health promotion and disease prevention, and collaboration with other healthcare providers and community organizations.

Mass casualty events, whether caused by natural disasters, terrorism, or other large-scale incidents, challenge the capacity of even the most robust emergency medical systems. Preparing for such events requires extensive planning, robust communication networks, and highly trained personnel. Paramedics play a vital role in triage, providing immediate medical care, and coordinating the transportation of victims to hospitals. Mass casualty incident (MCI) training is essential, encompassing various aspects, such as large-scale triage procedures, efficient resource management during chaos, and psychological support for both victims and responders. I've participated in numerous MCI drills and simulations, which have proven invaluable in honing our skills and coordinating responses under extreme pressure. However, these drills only partly prepare us for the emotional aftermath that can be even more devastating than the event itself.

Addressing these emerging public health challenges necessitates a multi-pronged strategy. Enhanced funding for EMS systems, continued investment in education and training, and the development of innovative technologies are critical. This also demands a closer collaboration between EMS, hospitals, and public health agencies to create a seamless and effective system. Data sharing, clear communication protocols, and integrated technologies will enhance response capacity and improve patient outcomes. The ability to quickly gather and analyze data during and after events will provide valuable insights for future preparedness efforts.

Furthermore, the integration of technology into paramedicine plays a growing role. Telemedicine allows paramedics to remotely consult with specialists, improving diagnosis and treatment, especially in rural and underserved areas. Wearable sensors and remote monitoring devices can provide real-time data on patient vital signs, enhancing early detection of deterioration. Advanced data analytics can help identify high-risk individuals and communities, allowing for targeted interventions. This advanced technological integration, while offering enormous potential, necessitates addressing concerns related to data security, privacy, and equitable access.

Finally, mental health support for paramedics is paramount. The inherent stressors of the job, combined with the increasing demands of public health challenges, take a significant toll on the mental and emotional well-being of paramedics. Access to mental health services, peer support programs, and robust organizational support are critical for maintaining a healthy and resilient paramedic workforce. This is not just a matter of individual well-being, but also a vital aspect of ensuring the continued effectiveness and reliability of emergency medical services. Investing in the mental health of paramedics is investing in the health and safety of our communities.

In conclusion, the future of paramedicine lies in adapting to and proactively addressing the growing complexities of public health. The evolution of the paramedic's role from simply responding to emergencies to proactively managing community health is crucial. This involves specialized training in disaster response, community health initiatives, and the ethical use of technology. Moreover, this necessitates a commitment to fostering resilience and providing comprehensive mental health support for the paramedics who remain on the front lines, bearing the brunt of these challenges, whilst maintaining compassion and excellence in the face of ever-increasing demands. The long-term health and safety of our communities hinge upon their ongoing dedication and well-being.

The evolving landscape of healthcare necessitates a corresponding evolution in the roles and responsibilities of paramedics. No longer confined to the traditional model of responding solely to emergency calls, paramedics are increasingly becoming integral components of comprehensive community healthcare systems. This expansion encompasses a wider range of duties, from preventative medicine and health education to advanced diagnostic capabilities and ongoing patient management.

One significant shift is the rise of community paramedicine programs. These initiatives leverage the unique skillset and accessibility of paramedics to address the growing burden of chronic diseases within communities. Instead of solely reacting to acute crises, paramedics are actively engaging in preventative care, conducting health screenings, delivering educational programs, and providing ongoing support for patients with chronic conditions like diabetes, hypertension, and heart failure. This proactive approach contributes to improved patient outcomes, reduced hospital readmissions, and a more efficient allocation of healthcare resources. I've witnessed firsthand the success of such programs in reducing hospital visits for patients with congestive heart failure, through regular check-ins, medication reconciliation, and early detection of complications. This approach not only improves the patient's quality of life but also eases the strain on overwhelmed emergency departments.

The expansion of paramedic scope of practice is another key trend. As healthcare systems grapple with shortages of physicians and other healthcare professionals, paramedics are being empowered to perform a broader range of medical procedures. This includes administering medications such as anticoagulants and administering advanced life support interventions, including cardiac monitoring and defibrillation. In rural and underserved areas where access to specialized medical care is limited, this expanded scope of practice is particularly crucial. The ability of paramedics to provide timely and effective care in such settings can be life-saving. Of course, this expanded scope necessitates rigorous training and ongoing professional development to ensure that paramedics possess the requisite skills and knowledge to perform these advanced procedures safely and effectively.

This enhanced responsibility also demands a heightened awareness of ethical considerations. Paramedics are increasingly called upon to make complex clinical decisions in challenging environments, often with limited resources and information. Ethical dilemmas related to resource allocation, end-of-life care, and patient autonomy must be addressed through comprehensive training and ongoing professional development. Ethical decision-making frameworks, coupled with opportunities for reflection and mentorship, are crucial to equip paramedics with the tools necessary to navigate these complex situations. One specific example that comes to mind involved a patient with end-stage cancer who repeatedly called for an ambulance due to worsening symptoms. Balancing the patient's desire for comfort and the efficient allocation of resources presented a difficult, though ultimately rewarding, ethical challenge.

The integration of technology is fundamentally reshaping the paramedic profession. Mobile data terminals provide access to real-time patient information, allowing for informed decision-making. Telemedicine platforms facilitate remote consultations with specialists, particularly valuable in remote areas or when specialized expertise is required. Wearable sensors and remote monitoring devices offer continuous monitoring of patients' vital signs, enabling early detection of changes in condition and facilitating proactive interventions. This technological integration demands robust data security protocols and training programs to ensure the responsible and ethical use of these technologies. I've seen personally the transformative potential of telemedicine in connecting patients in remote areas with specialists, bridging geographical barriers and ensuring access to high-quality care.

The increasing complexity of public health challenges further expands the paramedic's role. Addressing the growing prevalence of chronic diseases, managing the impact of climate change on health, and preparing for and responding to mass casualty incidents necessitate paramedics possessing advanced skills and training. Specialized training in disaster response, community health initiatives, and the ethical use of technology are paramount. Our role in responding to mass casualty events, whether natural disasters or other large-scale crises, necessitates detailed training in triage, rapid stabilization, resource management, and psychological support for both victims and responders. The mental and emotional toll of such events is significant, requiring robust support systems to mitigate long-term effects on both paramedics and communities.

Furthermore, the importance of mental health support for paramedics cannot be overstated. The inherent stressors of the job, coupled with the growing demands of public health challenges, place a considerable strain on the mental well-being of paramedics. Access to mental health services, peer support programs, and a culture of open communication and destigmatization are critical. Investing in the mental health of paramedics isn't merely an act of compassion but a vital investment in ensuring the continued effectiveness and resilience of the entire emergency medical services system. Without adequate support, burnout and compassion fatigue threaten the very fabric of this critical profession.

The future of paramedicine is undoubtedly one of continued expansion and evolution. The integration of community-based care, the expansion of scope of practice, the integration of technology, and a renewed focus on mental health support will be defining characteristics of the profession in the years to come. As paramedics embrace these evolving roles and responsibilities, they will become even more indispensable members of healthcare systems worldwide. This requires proactive investment in education, training, and support systems to enable paramedics to meet the complex demands of a rapidly changing healthcare landscape. The challenges are significant, but the potential to positively impact community health and improve patient outcomes is immense. The dedication, skill, and adaptability of paramedics are crucial, and continued investment in their professional growth is essential to secure a brighter future for both the profession and the communities they serve. The future of paramedicine is bright, but only if we invest in the people who are at the heart of it. The responsibility lies with us, as a profession and as a society, to ensure that those on the front lines have the tools and support they need to continue providing exemplary care.

Predicting the future is always a risky endeavor, particularly in a field as dynamic as paramedicine. However, by extrapolating from current trends and emerging technologies, we can paint a plausible picture of the paramedic profession in 2030 and beyond. One thing is certain: the role of the paramedic will continue to evolve, demanding adaptability, innovation, and a commitment to lifelong learning.

One of the most significant shifts we can expect is an even greater integration of paramedics into broader healthcare systems. The current movement toward community paramedicine will undoubtedly accelerate. We'll likely see paramedics taking on expanded roles in managing chronic conditions, conducting preventative health initiatives, and acting as liaisons between patients and healthcare providers. This will involve increasingly sophisticated data analysis, allowing paramedics to identify at-risk individuals and intervene proactively. Imagine a future where predictive algorithms, fed by data from wearable sensors and electronic health records, allow paramedics to identify patients at high risk for heart failure exacerbation days before a crisis occurs, allowing for timely interventions to prevent hospitalizations. This proactive approach will require significant investment in data infrastructure, training in data analysis, and the development of appropriate ethical guidelines to protect patient privacy. The ethical considerations of using predictive algorithms in healthcare are significant and warrant careful consideration.

The integration of advanced technology will continue to revolutionize paramedic practice. We've already seen the introduction of telemedicine, allowing remote consultations with specialists. However, the future will likely see the widespread adoption of artificial intelligence (AI) in various aspects of paramedic care. AI-powered diagnostic tools could assist paramedics in making more accurate and timely diagnoses in the field, reducing delays in treatment and improving patient outcomes. For instance, AI could analyze electrocardiograms (ECGs) in real time, identifying subtle abnormalities that might be missed by the human eye, potentially saving lives. This requires a careful consideration of the role of AI: will it supplement or replace human judgment? How will we ensure the accuracy and reliability of AI diagnostic tools? How will we address potential biases embedded in these systems? These are crucial questions that need to be addressed.

The expansion of the paramedic scope of practice will also be a major factor shaping the profession's future. We can anticipate paramedics taking on more advanced roles, potentially performing procedures currently reserved for physicians or nurses. This expanded scope of practice will necessitate significant investment in education and training to ensure paramedics possess the requisite skills and knowledge. Rigorous competency assessments and continuous professional development programs will be essential to guarantee the highest standards of safety and quality of care. This also raises important questions about licensing, regulation, and professional liability. As paramedics undertake more advanced procedures, the legal and ethical frameworks governing their practice will need to adapt to accommodate these changes. We'll need robust systems to monitor and review the outcomes of expanded scopes of practice to ensure continuous improvement and patient safety.

The demands on paramedics will only intensify in the coming years. The aging population, combined with increasing rates of chronic diseases, will result in a higher volume of emergency calls and a greater need for community-based care. Preparing for and responding to mass casualty incidents, whether natural disasters or large-scale terrorist events, will also require increasingly specialized training and enhanced coordination among emergency responders. The challenge will be to balance the increasing demands on the profession with ensuring the well-being of paramedics themselves. We cannot expect paramedics to continue operating at peak performance without adequate support for their mental and physical health.

This brings us to perhaps the most crucial aspect of the future of paramedicine: the urgent need for improved mental health support. The nature of the work – exposure to trauma, death, and suffering, combined with long hours, irregular shifts, and high-stakes decision-making – takes a significant toll on paramedics. The profession has a high rate of burnout and compassion fatigue, impacting not only individual well-being but also the quality of patient care. Investing in comprehensive mental health services, including access to counseling, peer support programs, and robust employee assistance programs, is not simply a matter of compassion; it is a vital investment in ensuring the long-term sustainability of the profession. Creating a culture of open communication, reducing stigma around mental health, and fostering a strong sense of community within paramedic teams are essential steps toward mitigating these challenges. This involves educating not only paramedics but also administrators and policymakers about the importance of mental health and fostering an environment that supports help-seeking behavior.

Finally, the future of paramedicine will also depend on effective advocacy and collaboration. Paramedics need to actively participate in shaping the future of the profession, engaging in policy discussions, advocating for increased funding for education and training, and working collaboratively with other healthcare professionals to ensure seamless integration within broader healthcare systems. This collaborative approach extends beyond traditional healthcare settings. Working with community leaders, social workers, and other organizations will be vital to addressing the social determinants of health that significantly impact patient outcomes. Building stronger relationships with hospitals and other healthcare providers is critical to ensure smooth transitions of care and improved patient outcomes.

Looking ahead to 2030 and beyond, the paramedic profession faces both significant challenges and remarkable opportunities. The continuing evolution of technology, the expansion of scope of practice, and the increasing integration of paramedics into community-based healthcare systems will reshape the landscape of emergency medical services. However, success will hinge on a commitment to investing in the well-being of paramedics, fostering a culture of support, and ensuring access to comprehensive mental health resources. The future of paramedicine is bright, but only if we prioritize the health and well-being of those who bravely serve on the front lines, providing critical care to those in need. The commitment to lifelong learning, adapting to change, and embracing innovation will be crucial for ensuring the continued success and relevance of this vital profession. The future, therefore, depends not only on technological advancements but also on a holistic approach that recognizes and values the human element at the heart of paramedicine.

This appendix provides a curated collection of resources to support paramedics in navigating the emotional, physical, and professional challenges of their demanding careers. It is divided into three sections: Mental Health Resources, Coping Mechanisms and Stress Management Techniques, and Career Transition Resources.

Section 1: Mental Health Resources for First Responders

The following organizations provide confidential support, crisis intervention, peer assistance, education, and mental-health resources specifically tailored to first responders. All contact information is current and verified.

1. Safe Call Now

Website: https://www.safecallnowusa.org

Phone (24/7): 1-206-459-3020

Alternate Line: 1-877-230-6060

About:

A confidential crisis line staffed by active and retired public-safety professionals. Provides immediate peer support for first responders and their families, along with referrals to vetted mental health services.

2. COPLINE – Confidential Support Line for Law Enforcement

Website: https://copline.org

Phone (24/7): 1-800-267-5463

About:

A 24-hour hotline answered by trained, retired law-enforcement officers. Offers emotional support, crisis de-escalation, and guidance for active or retired officers facing job-related stress, trauma, or personal struggles.

3. National Suicide & Crisis Lifeline (988)

Website: https://988lifeline.org

Call/Text: 988

Chat: Available through website

About:

A nationwide crisis line accessible by phone, text, or chat. First responders can use the service anonymously for immediate support, crisis intervention, or connection to local mental-health resources.

4. National Volunteer Fire Council – "Share the Load" Program

Website: https://www.nvfc.org/help

Fire/EMS Helpline (24/7): 1-888-731-FIRE (3473)

About:

A confidential support program for firefighters, EMS personnel, and their families. Provides phone support, educational resources, training, and referrals for behavioral health services.

5. The Quell Foundation – First Responder Resilience Project

Website: https://quellfrrp.org/resources

Crisis Text Line: Text **741741**

Fire/EMS Helpline: 1-844-525-3473

General Crisis Number: 988

About:

A dedicated resource hub for first responder mental health. Offers resilience tools, crisis contacts, research-based guidance, and connections to first-responder-specific therapy and support networks.

6. NAMI – Public Safety Professionals Support Resources

Website:
https://www.nami.org/your-journey/frontline-professionals/public-safety-professionals/peer-support-resources

NAMI HelpLine: 1-800-950-NAMI (6264)

Text Line: Text **"HELPLINE"** to **62640**

About:

Provides mental-health education, peer support groups, and resource navigation tailored to EMS, fire, dispatch, and law-enforcement personnel. Focuses on early intervention, coping strategies, and family support.

7. Crisis Text Line (General)

Website: https://www.crisistextline.org

Text: 741741

About:

A 24/7 text-based crisis service staffed by trained volunteer counselors. Ideal for responders who prefer silent communication or are unable to make voice calls during high-stress moments.

8. IAFF Center of Excellence (Fire/EMS)

Website: https://www.iaffrecoverycenter.com

Phone: 1-855-900-8437

About:

A treatment and recovery program specifically designed for firefighters and EMS personnel. Provides inpatient and outpatient care for PTSD, addiction, depression, and job-related trauma.

9. First Responder Support Network (FRSN)

Website: https://www.frsn.org

Phone: 1-415-721-9789

About:

Offers residential treatment programs, peer support, and workshops for first responders coping with trauma, cumulative stress, depression, or exposure-related mental health conditions.

10. EMS Professionals Peer Support Directory

Website:

https://www.naemt.org/initiatives/ems-mental-health-resources

About:

A national directory created by NAEMT to connect EMS workers with peer teams, mental-health clinicians, resiliency training, and organizational support systems.

Appendix – Example Coping Strategies for First Responders

The following strategies are commonly used by paramedics, EMTs, firefighters, law enforcement officers, and dispatchers to manage stress, regulate emotions, and reduce the impact of cumulative trauma. These can be adapted to fit individual needs and personal routines.

1. Grounding Techniques

- **4-6 Breathing:** Inhale for 4 seconds, exhale for 6 seconds; reduces sympathetic activation.
- **Sensory Reset:** Identify 5 things you can see, 4 you can touch, 3 you can hear, 2 you can smell, 1 you can taste.
- **Cold Stimulus:** Holding a cold bottle or using cold water can interrupt adrenaline spikes.

2. Physical Regulation

- **Post-Shift Walks:** 10–15 minutes helps metabolize stress hormones.
- **Stretching or Mobility Work:** Reduces physical tension after long transports or heavy lifting.
- **Controlled Exercise:** Lifting, running, rowing, or yoga to discharge stored stress.

3. Mental and Emotional Processing

- **Call Decompression:** Talking through a tough call with a trusted partner, supervisor, or peer.
- **Narrative Writing:** Short journaling about what happened, what you felt, and what you learned.

- **Compartment Review:** Identifying what is yours to carry vs. what belongs to the job.

4. Sensory Reset After Difficult Calls

- **Music Therapy:** Use familiar playlists that signal "off duty" in the brain.
- **Shower Reset:** Warm shower followed by brief cool rinse to reduce cortisol.
- **Aromatherapy:** Simple scents like eucalyptus or lavender to down-shift the nervous system.

5. Connection and Support

- **Check-Ins with Partners or Friends:** Short, honest texts like "rough shift but okay."
- **Family Debrief Rules:** Set boundaries around what you share, when, and how.
- **Peer Support Groups:** Connecting with others who understand without needing long explanations.

6. Slow-Down Strategies After High-Adrenaline Calls

- **10-Minute Rule:** Don't go straight to bed or straight home after a critical call; decompress first.
- **Hydration and Light Food:** Replenish after adrenaline spikes; prevents headaches and fatigue.
- **Soft Tasks:** Folding laundry, cleaning rigs, organizing gear—simple, grounding tasks.

7. Long-Term Wellness Habits

- **Regular Therapy:** Preferably with someone specializing in first responders or trauma.
- **Consistent Sleep Routine:** Target same sleep/wake windows whenever possible.
- **Healthy Boundaries:** Learning to say "I'm off shift" and meaning it.
- **Skill Refreshers:** Keeping clinical confidence high reduces anticipatory anxiety.

8. Creative and Personal Outlets

- **Hobbies:** Woodworking, gaming, writing, painting—anything that shifts focus away from work.
- **Nature Time:** Parks, forests, beaches, or stargazing to regulate the nervous system.
- **Mindful Activities:** Puzzles, cooking, handcrafts, or anything requiring gentle focus.

9. Crisis / High-Stress Moment Tools

- **Call a hotline or peer support line** from your appendix resources.
- **Crisis Text Line (741741):** Fast, quiet help in moments of overload.
- **Buddy Check:** Reach out to your closest peer when something feels "off."

10. Off-Shift Rituals

- **Transition Routine:** Remove uniform, shower, hydrate, change clothes, then "enter home."
- **Night Reset:** Quiet room, low light, reduce stimulants, calming audio.
- **Positive Anchor:** Spend 2–5 minutes on something that reminds you why you still care about the job.

Good Resources for Paramedic Career Transition

Resource / Program	What It Offers / How It Helps
National Association of Emergency Medical Technicians (NAEMT)	Offers certifications, continuing-education courses, and a network to leverage EMS skills into related health or safety careers.
International Association of Fire Fighters (IAFF) / Center of Excellence	Offers support services for EMS/firefighters looking to shift roles — this can include training, mental-health wraparound support, or career counseling when leaving field duty.
NAMI & First Responder Mental Health Peer Directories	Useful if you want to transition into peer support, counselor-adjacent, or wellness / advocacy roles — helps with training and networking.
Community College / University EMS-to-Health Degrees (e.g. Nursing, Physician Assistant, Paramedic-to-RN bridge)	Many paramedic skills transfer; shorter bridge programs allow licensure or schooling for other medical careers.

Resource / Program	What It Offers / How It Helps
Local EMS agencies offering "crossover" or "retraining" for Fire, Rescue, OR non-transport EMS teams	Using your EMS license/training, you can shift to other public-safety or medical-support roles (fire, rescue, transport, tactical EMS).
Peer networks / mentorship groups for ex-medics & first responders	Many former medics share transition paths publicly — helpful for real-world insight, support, and advice when shifting careers.

◈ *Practical Transition Paths for Paramedics*

- **Paramedic → Registered Nurse (RN)**: With bridging or accelerated nursing programs; EMS experience is strong background.

- **Paramedic → Physician Assistant (PA) or Nurse Practitioner (NP)**: Long-term education needed, but EMS gives a solid foundation in acute care, diagnostics, triage, and patient interaction.

- **Paramedic → Fire / Rescue Personnel**: If you want to stay in public safety but shift away from transport calls.

- **Paramedic → EMS Instructor / Training Coordinator**: Teaching future medics, leading continuing education, shaping EMS protocols.

- **Paramedic → Occupational Health / Safety, Industrial Medic, Tactical Medic**: Applying EMS training to private-sector safety, security teams, or corporate first response.

- **Paramedic → Peer Support / Mental-Health Advocate for First Responders**: Drawing on field experience and personal insight to help others cope with stress, trauma, and burnout.

- **Paramedic → Healthcare Administration / Case Management / Dispatch / Logistics**: Non-frontline roles using EMS knowledge but less intense environment.

Steven "Mork" Morken is a seasoned paramedic with nearly two decades on the front lines of emergency medicine. His career has spanned 911 response, theme-park health services, and high-acuity clinical care, giving him a grounded, no-nonsense view of what it truly means to serve others under pressure. Known for his clarity, compassion, and steady presence, he blends clinical expertise with real-world insight to help readers understand, survive, and navigate the demands of modern EMS.

Mork is the founder of **Morken Marketing LLC**, where he creates practical guides, mental health tools, and educational resources for first responders. His writing focuses on resilience, emotional survival, and the reality of life behind the uniform. He draws from his extensive certifications, field experience, and personal journey through trauma, recovery, and leadership growth.

When he isn't writing, he enjoys woodworking, gaming, and stargazing with his family in Florida. His long-term dream is simple, quiet, and honest, rooted in the same values that shape his books: build a life with intention, help others grow, and never lose sight of the bigger picture.